CALM
YOUR MIND
WITH
FOOD

Also by Uma Naidoo, MD

This Is Your Brain on Food: An Indispensable Guide to the Surprising Foods That Fight Depression, Anxiety, PTSD, OCD, ADHD, and More

CALM
YOUR MIND
WITH
FOOD

A REVOLUTIONARY GUIDE TO CONTROLLING YOUR ANXIETY

UMA NAIDOO, MD

Little, Brown Spark
New York Boston London

Copyright © 2023 by Uma Naidoo

Hachette Book Group supports the right to free expression and the value of copyright. The purpose of copyright is to encourage writers and artists to produce the creative works that enrich our culture.

The scanning, uploading, and distribution of this book without permission is a theft of the author's intellectual property. If you would like permission to use material from the book (other than for review purposes), please contact permissions@hbgusa.com. Thank you for your support of the author's rights.

Little, Brown Spark
Hachette Book Group
1290 Avenue of the Americas, New York, NY 10104
littlebrownspark.com

First Edition: December 2023

Little, Brown Spark is an imprint of Little, Brown and Company, a division of Hachette Book Group, Inc. The Little, Brown Spark name and logo are trademarks of Hachette Book Group, Inc.

The publisher is not responsible for websites (or their content) that are not owned by the publisher.

The Hachette Speakers Bureau provides a wide range of authors for speaking events. To find out more, go to hachettespeakersbureau.com or email HachetteSpeakers@hbgusa.com.

Little, Brown and Company books may be purchased in bulk for business, educational, or promotional use. For information, please contact your local bookseller or the Hachette Book Group Special Markets Department at special.markets@hbgusa.com.

ISBN 9780316502092
LCCN 2023941627

Printing 1, 2023

LSC-C

Printed in the United States of America

This book is dedicated to my parents, who instilled in me that education was my way to rise above apartheid and attain freedom, something they never had. And to my spouse, who is my biggest, boldest cheerleader.

Contents

Contents

Part III: The Protocol

CALM
YOUR MIND
WITH
FOOD

Introduction

My first book came out at a difficult time. A publication date of August 2020 meant that a carefully planned rollout was totally wrecked during the height of the COVID-19 pandemic. The situation in the world was evolving so rapidly that it took some time for virtual book tours and remote keynote talks to solidify, and I was left to worry that my work to communicate the importance of nutritional psychiatry would go unnoticed. Dwarfing that worry was the stress of being a frontline physician during such a terrifyingly uncertain time.

Thanks to the heroic efforts of my amazing publication team, my book launch didn't sputter as I feared it would. The pandemic brought additional attention to both mental health and food—after all, many of us were left with nothing to do but eat and worry, worry and eat. As the book found success, I should have been delighted about how it was helping people around the world better understand the relationship between the food they eat and the inner workings of their brain. But though I felt grateful that people were reading and learning from the book, the burden of those early days of the pandemic didn't lift. If anything, it got heavier. Strange as it may seem, with every accolade, news feature, TV appearance, and positive review, I felt a huge panic about what was next. Thinking about how to keep the momentum going wasn't exciting and fulfilling; it was scary. I felt like I couldn't do it.

As a psychiatrist who has spent years diagnosing anxiety in others, I know how to recognize the signs. I had felt them before too, when I was diagnosed with cancer and facing a daunting schedule of chemotherapy and other treatments. That was my first obvious struggle with my own mental health, and when I experienced the true power of nutritional psychiatry. Food helped me ease my anxiety and support my medical treatment, which provided the blueprint of my work today.

But this felt different. Instead of staring down a deadly disease, I was being invited to be a guest on television programs and podcasts, becoming colleagues and friends with some of my medical and media heroes, like Deepak Chopra. When I made myself step back and gain some perspective, I knew I should feel lucky and elated and grateful. But somehow the overwhelm and anxiety were the emotions that prevailed. To complicate matters further, despite paying attention to my food and finding time to exercise, I began to gain weight, due in part to stress and anxiety, but also to the aftermath of chemotherapy wreaking havoc on my metabolism. Though I fought with my self-consciousness, I could not shake the feeling that gaining weight somehow undermined my points about healthy nutrition, which further compounded my anxiety about appearances and talks.

As time went by, it seemed like nothing was working. My usual self-care practices, mindful eating, meditation, yoga, and other forms of exercise all felt like drops in an ocean of anxiety. I worked hard to keep my nutrition consistent, but the way I was feeling was like I had gone on a French fries–and–doughnuts regimen. At times, my anxiety bubbled up over these ongoing issues and I felt totally hopeless, stopping exercise for days and then losing track of my nutrition. Worries about the pandemic along with everything else disrupted my sleep, as coronasomnia reared its head. Everything combined into a cycle of angst, stress, and anxiety that continued to feed itself.

When it came time to start planning a new book, I immediately knew what subject I wanted to write about: anxiety. The world's most diagnosed mental health condition had arrived on my doorstep, and I hoped that by learning more about the cutting-edge research into the connections between nutrition and anxiety, I would be able to both help myself manage my own anxiety and shed light on such an urgent and complicated topic for others. Through my clinical work and my research for the first book, I already knew about how intertwined anxiety was with the gut microbiome, but as I started compiling articles and drafting the earliest parts of this book, I found myself taken aback at how anxiety is tied in with so many different aspects of physical health, including immunity, inflammation, leptin response, and metabolism.

This research made me grapple with the deeper layers of what anxiety does to the body and brain. Studying how tightly anxiety is connected to metabolic disruption gave me some insight into how my anxiety had helped make my metabolism go awry, leading to my stubborn weight gain. And learning about how anxiety is interlinked with the appetite hormone leptin gave me a basis for understanding why my anxiety had caused me to wolf down my meals but somehow left me less satiated even though I was eating more. This was a painful reminder that even healthy foods can be harmful when they aren't eaten in moderation.

Working on the book gave me the fortitude to redouble my efforts to take small steps toward quashing my anxiety, trusting that the sum of small, simple actions would have a big effect on how I was feeling. Once they were allowed under COVID restrictions, I booked regular massages and other spa treatments to help alleviate stress. I discovered a fun type of squeezable scented clay that I carried in my purse when I traveled to use as a stress ball when things were feeling tense. I chose a relaxing lavender and a soothing ocean scent, since the ocean has always been a calming place for me. (You can find my recipe for homemade Lavender Play Dough on page 270.) I relearned alternate nostril breathing, a yogic breath exercise that calms and relaxes, and began to practice it daily. I went to see a Transcendental Meditation teacher to sharpen my skills, which had been feeling dull. Since I had felt disconnected from yoga, I learned qigong, an ancient Chinese movement practice that gently involves the whole body, with the goal of lowering inflammation in the brain and body. Eventually, I was able to restart my morning sun salutation yoga, which I'd always used to welcome the day with positive energy.

To stem the tide of a seemingly endless set of obligations and appearances, I invested in a time management system for my iPad, which helped me organize my relentlessly busy days. I began to push back on deadlines proposed by media for submitting a quote or an article, and I began to agree to appear on podcasts only on days that worked well for my busy hospital schedule.

As for my diet, I cut back from 3 cups of coffee per day to 1 and gently increased the amount of water I was drinking to offset dehydration, which can worsen anxiety. I updated my beloved grandmother's golden chai recipe by adding more anxiety-relieving spices, and I made a point to drink it every day. This helped ground me in a positive childhood memory, as well as providing my brain with healing bioactive phytochemicals. Along with reminding myself to eat mindfully and chew my food slowly, I recognized I may have a form of leptin resistance and began to address that through stress management and my food choices. While I did not restrict calories, I was careful not to eat the French fries or other unhealthy choices my friends or family ordered when we were able to eat together again. I leaned into cruciferous vegetables, which are satiating and help offset the hunger pangs that an imbalanced appetite hormone can create. I ate as many leafy greens as I could—both for salads and for a nourishing smoothie on my workout days. I began to carry a healthy nut mix in case I was hungry and came across a tempting doughnut! I urged myself to get back in touch with my love of cooking, developing some of the recipes that appear in this book and finding some new favorite foods like the purple sprouting broccoli that is pictured on the cover.

The combination of these anxiety-lowering techniques did help me feel more grounded, and I regained the ability to live in the moment and focus on the task at hand. But I still didn't feel quite whole until I experienced two different, personal events.

Though I have always worked hard in my own therapy to shed the anxiety surrounding my experience with cancer, I didn't quite understand how deeply it was rooted in my unconscious. Several times each year, I went in for my tests and exams. In the middle of writing this book, I went in as usual for one such checkup. As she looked over the results, my doctor looked at me and said, "I've got great news; your tests are normal and we're graduating you out of the follow-up clinic and into the survivorship clinic." I looked at her with surprise and elation but simultaneously teared up. As I tearfully thanked her, I felt as though a massive weight had been physically lifted off my shoulders. My heart slowed to a normal pace, my breathing became more regular, and as I stood up, I felt light and free.

When you've lived through an illness like cancer, you wake up every day after your initial diagnosis wondering if you will survive. At first, it's a conscious and visceral worry. As you persevere through stages of care and treatment, it lessens in volume, but it persists as something you live with every time you take a breath. You move through your day and your life, and over time perhaps you learn to ignore it, but it remains beneath the surface. Hearing my doctor say those words freed me from mental shackles that I'd gotten so used to that I barely understood they were there. The tightly wound screw in my chest was loosening, and daylight somehow seemed brighter. That evening something changed when I ate dinner. I was less hungry, but food tasted better. I was able to eat slowly and mindfully and had no trouble understanding when I was full.

As I moved through those next few days feeling significantly calmer, I had a chance meeting that provided another crucial bit of understanding to help free me from anxiety. I was meeting a friend for dinner, and she asked if she could bring along a healer who had really helped her. I was a bit skeptical, but my reduction in anxiety after getting my good news made me feel more open to new and different experiences. As it turned out, he and I took to each other almost instantaneously. As we spoke over dinner, he deduced something profound about my life, my background, and my trauma—something I have always kept well hidden.

I grew up in South Africa under apartheid. While apartheid policies that separated whites and Blacks are well-known, Indian families were also kept separate, living under inferior conditions. As a child, I could not go to the same playgrounds or amusement parks as my white peers, and I had to attend separate schools that were subpar compared to white facilities. I don't think I truly understood what that meant at the time—I'm not sure a child truly can understand such naked hatred and prejudice. But the healer was able to piercingly see into my soul and mobilize some emotions I had never been able to fully form before. When you grow up in a society that judges your every action by your skin color, you develop a deep sense of shame. You try to hide yourself. It made me feel like success would lead to being targeted and it was safer to hide. Even though I was valedictorian in school, captain of my sports team, a ballet dancer, and a pianist, it seemed like my accomplishments meant little, superseded by my skin color. My proud parents kept an album of my many award certificates, trophies, and medals, but to white South African society, I was of no consequence.

I slowly began to understand this same feeling was at the root of my current struggles with anxiety too. It was a humbling reminder of the complexity of the human mind. While those around me cheered on my book and my work, a painful hollowness lingered inside. But for the first time, it seemed as though I could bring that hollow feeling to the surface and make it whole. Sometimes it takes a bold person who leaps in and calls out a problem, bringing it to conscious attention.

Understanding and relieving myself of the burdens from my experience with cancer and my childhood trauma gave me the final tool to unlock my anxiety and metabolic struggles. The pressures of a successful book and the fears of living through a global pandemic both felt clearer and more possible to navigate with my new outlook. And finally, I was able to help my metabolism reset as I cleared the way to ease my anxiety. I was returned to my normal weight and once more felt that I could enjoy life without the looming specter of worry.

All of this is to say that I wrote this book out of concern and compassion for my patients and professional curiosity about an exciting and engaging field of science, but I also wrote it out of the pain of personal experience. I was seeing more anxiety every day in my clinical work, reading about it on the news, seeing more suicides being reported than ever before in my career. But I was living the struggle too. Mental well-being is for everyone; anxiety doesn't discriminate, and it can affect any one of us. The ability to fight against anxiety should not be reserved only for those who have access to good health care. We need more accessible solutions that don't require prescriptions and insurance. Food and nutrition are valuable tools that can get us many steps closer to relieving anxiety, alongside other treatments and breakthroughs. Eating is something every person must do every day. We cannot afford to neglect such a basic way to strive for good mental health.

If you are feeling anxious, you are not alone. In this book, we will learn how fundamentally anxiety is connected with your brain and body, and how you can harness the power at the end of your fork to calm your mind with food.

PART I: THE PROBLEM

CHAPTER ONE

Fighting the Global Anxiety Epidemic

W hile writing this book, I was invited to give a keynote lecture at the first Integrative and Personalised Medicine conference in London. It was a huge honor to be asked to speak at an international conference, and I was delighted that the event's leadership was interested in my work. I humbly accepted, feeling confident about presenting to a group of like-minded clinicians. It can certainly be nerve-wracking to speak in front of a group of doctors—especially in person after a few years of acclimating to video chat—but I have enough experience in similar situations that I trusted my ability to stay calm and professional.

What followed nearly caused me to faint. I received an email informing me that my work had gained the attention of the royal family. Along with three other American doctors, I was invited to meet His Royal Highness the Prince of Wales—who has since become the king of England—to discuss our work. It had to be a mistake. I was going to meet Prince Charles? How on earth could this even happen?

The anxiety I'd brushed off from the original invitation flooded over me like a gushing fire hydrant. My palms were sweating, my thoughts raced, and my heart pounded in my chest. The impostor syndrome I've spent years fighting reared its head. Surely the Prince of Wales would see through me. It would be the end of my career! My anxious brain distorted what should have been such a positive moment into something completely different.

Thankfully, I was able to wrest control of my feelings. I couldn't let anxiety create failure. I focused myself on the moment and did some exercises from pranayama, or breath work yoga. It took me time to settle down and be able to fully accept the situation, but by the time I typed out a measured and courteous "yes" to the invitation, I felt calm, making space for excitement and joy.

Once I was in London, as my meeting with the prince approached, I had to actively work on separating my excitement from my fear and anxiety. The morning of the event, I woke up early, meditated, and made sure to drink cool water, which helps relieve any overnight dehydration; and the coolness always feels calming for my brain and body. I ate a breakfast full of calming foods, like tofu scramble seasoned with turmeric and black pepper, with mushrooms and spinach on the side. I managed to stay calm and focused when my roller hairbrush shorted out, even though the prospect of a bad hair day has always been a mood ruiner for me. As I planned out my dress and practiced my curtsy, I did more breath work and used mindfulness to keep my thoughts from spiraling. Even though I went to the meeting with some butterflies in my stomach, the worst of my anxiety had subsided, and I could walk in with confidence.

You can probably guess how the meeting went. Prince Charles was lovely, as were the other doctors present, and we had a lively discussion about the kind of whole-body approach to mental health that we will learn about in this book. It was not the end of my career, but the amazing start to an exciting role as the US ambassador for the UK College of Medicine, leading the Food for Mood Campaign.

On the plane home from the United Kingdom, I reflected on how anxiety had nearly derailed such a game-changing moment in my life. It can be easy to minimize anxious feelings, telling yourself to *toughen up* or *get over it*. Nevertheless, anxiety is real and damaging. I was thankful that I had been able to calm my anxiety through a combination of practice, an understanding of how the brain works, and a diet that creates a strong foundation for mental health. It made me think of my patients who've had similar struggles, whether with specific challenges in their lives and careers or with the kind of pervasive anxiety that seizes on the smallest details to throw their worlds into chaos.

The whole experience was a powerful reminder of how grateful I am to have the opportunity to help others improve their mental health and understand and overcome their anxiety through the powerful medicine of food.

THE ANXIETY EPIDEMIC

The American Psychiatric Association (APA) conducts a variety of public opinion polls, including a recent monthly poll called Healthy Minds Monthly, which provide a fascinating window into the mental health of the average American.[1] Looking through poll results from the past few years highlights growing concerns about a litany of stressors both modern and timeless: the effects of social media, the health and safety of our children, workplace stress, and the ability to make ends meet. In March 2020, anxiety was boosted into overdrive by the sudden rise of COVID-19, with 48 percent of Americans reporting anxiety about catching the novel disease, and even greater numbers worried about it harming their loved ones, their finances, and the overall economy.[2] But as COVID-specific anxiety began to recede, it was quickly replaced by worries about returning to the workplace, the war in Ukraine, climate change, inflation, and the specter of mass shootings.[3] In October 2022, 79 percent of adults said that the state of mental health in the United States was a public health emergency.[4]

The APA's findings are just one piece in a deluge of evidence that we are experiencing an unprecedented anxiety crisis. Anxiety is the most commonly diagnosed mental health condition in the world, with our best epidemiological surveys showing that up to 33.7 percent of people will suffer from an anxiety disorder in their life-time.[5] Other estimates show that around 40 million Americans, or 18.1 percent of the population, suffer from anxiety every year.[6] We know that anxiety tends to be more prevalent in women than men,[7] and that disparities in access to health care can pose a par-ticular challenge to treating anxiety in communities of color.[8] Espe-cially troubling is skyrocketing anxiety in young people. Between 2016 and 2020, anxiety diagnoses in children ages three to seven-teen increased 29 percent.[9] Anxiety is so common among all groups that in September 2022, the US Preventive Services Task Force recommended that all adults under sixty-five be screened for anxiety.[10]

If you're reading this book, I suspect you have firsthand knowl-edge about anxiety's destructive power, or perhaps you've seen it eat away at a loved one. You are likely familiar with the racing thoughts, sweaty palms, and nausea that can leave you feeling unable to get out of bed and face the day. But as serious as the day-to-day mental symptoms of anxiety can be, they don't tell the whole story. Anxiety can put you at greater risk for heart disease,[11] diabetes,[12] autoimmune conditions,[13] and Alzheimer's.[14] As a cancer survivor myself, I have direct experience with how anxiety can hit you like a six-ton truck barreling down the Massachusetts Turnpike, complicating the body's recovery from serious disease.

Perhaps most insidiously, anxiety tends to feed on itself. In my patients, I often see how worries compound one another, one stressor feeding into another until their mental health is sent into a down-ward spiral. I'm certainly susceptible to that as well—even research-ing and writing out these statistics, my heart rate is elevated and my palms are sweaty. But when I step away from the screen and take a deep breath and a mindfulness moment, I remember that despite the colossal challenge of the global anxiety crisis, it's not time for despair. While it can feel dizzying to consider the numbers of people suffering from anxiety across the globe, as a psychiatrist, I am heartened by our growing knowledge of the intricate workings of the human brain and our understanding about how good mental health is a team effort that requires support from across your body. As a nutritional psychiatrist, I'm thrilled by the evidence that proves that food can be an indispensable tool in improving mental health. And as a chef, I love to envision the creativity and flair with which home cooks can combine healthy ingredients into delicious, nourishing, anxiety-busting meals.

Even during an unprecedented anxiety crisis, our knowledge about this condition is rapidly increasing, with particularly massive strides being made in our understanding of how anxiety is not just a mental condition but a complex, interlinked illness that has to be treated with a full-body approach. In this book, we will dig into the latest research about the ways anxiety is rooted in our brain, our gut, our immune system, and our metabolism, all of which have to be functioning properly to keep our minds calm and clear.

WHAT IS ANXIETY?

Human emotions are complex. The most even-keeled person in the world is still buffeted by the winds of emotion, experiencing joyous highs and dismal lows — sometimes in rapid succession. My meeting with the Prince of Wales should have been a proud and affirming prospect, but instead my mind retreated into roiling anxiety. Why?

The study of emotion is called affective science, and it's one of the most exciting and groundbreaking psychiatric fields of study. Long-held hypotheses about what is going on in the brain as different emotions are triggered are being called into question as new theories arise. Even with our growing breadth of knowledge about mental health, we do not have a clear understanding of exactly what causes anxiety, but we do know that many factors play a role. In the biopsychosocial model of anxiety, we classify the factors as:

- Biological: genetics, neurochemistry (for instance, neurotransmitter imbalances), health conditions, chronic disease, and nutritional factors

- Psychological: personality traits, anxiety sensitivity, history of trauma

- Social: loneliness, sleep quality, exercise, substance abuse[15]

For a given individual, any of these factors may weigh more heavily than the others, and different people can respond in different ways to the same set of stressors. Scenarios that might cause extreme anxiety in one person might feel totally routine to others. And an anxiety-fighting strategy that works well for one person may not get the same results in others. It's all part of the confounding, enigmatic puzzle of the human brain.

Regardless of what specific factors lead to anxiety, it sparks a distinct set of unconscious physiological processes in your body. To understand how your body reacts to anxiety, it's helpful to first understand its cousin, fear. Fear is a primal and visceral emotion brought on by the presence of real danger. When you detect danger through one of your five senses, a small part of your brain called the amygdala is activated, spreading the alarm to the nearby hypothalamus. The hypothalamus is tightly connected to your pituitary and adrenal glands in a relationship called the hypothalamic-pituitary-adrenal axis (HPA-axis), which releases hormones like adrenaline and cortisol and coordinates with your autonomic nervous system (ANS) to trigger a fight-or-flight response.

The combined effect of this cascading fear response is that your senses are heightened to help you respond to the threat. For instance, if you're driving and you see that six-ton truck crossing into your lane, your HPA-axis and ANS will spring into action. Your heart rate will increase, your pupils and blood vessels will dilate, you'll breathe more heavily, and your body will make extra energy available to your cells. With these heightened powers, your brain and body are better able to react quickly enough that you can swerve to the side and avoid a potentially fatal crash.

It's easy to see why the fear response is useful — even essential — to our ability to survive in a dangerous world. It also feels intuitive that it would be hardwired into our brain's circuitry — if our ancestors had been less inclined to feel fear, their genes might not have survived, thanks to natural selection. After all, it's not just humans who experience a fear response — we see similar feelings at work in animals every time a squirrel flees from an overeager dog.

Fear is a subset of a broader category of physiological reactions called the stress response. In everyday life, we generally think of stress as being psychological or emotional strain from difficulties with family, work, school, finances, or other everyday challenges. However, in medical terminology, stress has a more inclusive definition; one study describes it as "any intrinsic or extrinsic stimulus that evokes a biological response."[16] By that definition, the truck crossing into your lane is a stressor, but so is the worry brought on by having to make a presentation at work. Though these scenarios pose different levels of threat, both elicit the same basic response in your body, igniting your amygdala and triggering a cascade of stress response via the HPA-axis and ANS. That's why you might feel similar feelings of panic, jumpiness, excessive sweating, and increased heart rate, whether you're in imminent danger or you're simply nervous about a task that is looming over you. While the intensity of the stress response may vary, the basic pathways are the same.

While stress and anxiety are linked, there is a crucial difference between the two. The stress response is caused by active stimuli that your body is reacting to. Ideally, when the stressor is removed, the stress response dissipates, and your body can return to normal function. Anxiety, on the other hand, is concerned with the future, anticipating potential threats that have not yet materialized. Our brains are wired to be on constant alert for the possibility of trouble, always vigilantly looking out for our well-being. That's a good thing, at least in moderation, and it forms another important part of our natural defense system, allowing us to anticipate threats and keep ourselves out of danger. But it's easy for our brains to tip over into being unreasonable about the dangers we face, imagining threats that aren't there, or overestimating the seriousness of the ones that are. We might be anxious about getting into a car crash or contracting a life-threatening illness like COVID-19, but anxiety can be equally debilitating when it's about work, family, or social situations. My meeting with Prince Charles certainly wasn't putting me in any kind of tangible danger, but that didn't stop my anxiety from bounding to the irrational idea that this great opportunity would somehow lead to my professional downfall.

Regardless of the source of our anxiety, these feelings lock our brain into unnecessary patterns of stress response, hogging our mind's and body's precious resources, causing a host of cognitive and physical symptoms like poor concentration, racing thoughts, confusion, elevated heart rate, dizziness, and upset stomach. The same thought pathways and physiological responses that might help us survive in a split-second life-or-death scenario become an unnecessary weight on our brains and bodies, robbing us of healthy mental function. And since anxiety is so difficult to treat, it's common for people to suffer from it for long periods of time—months, years, or even their whole lives. The burden from living in a constant state of stress response brought on by anxiety can cause or worsen a host of serious medical conditions, including a weakened immune system, chronic inflammation, and an increased risk of metabolic disorders like type 2 diabetes.

THE THEORY OF CONSTRUCTED EMOTION

Modern affective science has opened up new pathways to understanding the basis of emotions, including fear and anxiety. For instance, Lisa Feldman Barrett, a neuroscientist I respect and admire, has challenged the idea that emotions are hardwired into our brains by thousands of years of evolution. Through extensive research on facial, physiological, and neural responses to emotion, she has developed a new school of thought called "the theory of constructed emotion," which posits that emotions are "built" in the brain.[17] Rather than relying on an innate circuitry of response to threats, Barrett proposes that our brains are constantly assembling predictions about the world around us, based on our previous experience. Instead of being a hardwired and universal reaction to a threat, she argues that fear is, in essence, a learned behavior, a result of our brain's constant search for ways to understand and contextualize the world.

The theory of constructed emotion represents a paradigm shift in affective science, with profound implications across the spectrum of how we understand human nature. But most important for our purposes, it sheds light on the source of anxiety. Rather than a primal anticipation of tangible threat in our animal brain, to Barrett, anxiety is instead a predictive response that our brain draws from our past experience. When an anxiety-provoking situation causes us to panic, it's because we have prepared our brains to panic.

When faced with the idea of meeting Prince Charles to talk about my work, my brain raced to construct emotions surrounding the possibility of meeting a powerful person, jumping straight to anxiety about everything that could go wrong, even though there was no logical threat. What if I could have stopped preparing for anxiety and replaced it with excitement or happiness instead? Barrett's theory provides room for doing just that, retraining the brain to construct positive rather than negative emotions. This might seem like wishful thinking if you've struggled with anxiety your whole life. But guess what: anxiety is only one of many configurations under which your brain can operate. You can change this configuration by thinking in different ways. Reframing, distraction, acceptance, and mindfulness have all been shown to tamp down anxiety or, in the best of circumstances, change your brain's predictive response from "anxious" to "excited" or "present."[18] As Barrett explains in her popular TED talk, you aren't at the mercy of your emotions.[19] While Barrett's work is geared toward fighting anxiety through mental strategies, and mine is focused on calming your mind through food, we both agree that you have more control than you think.

While Barrett's theory has tantalizing possibilities for strategies to treat anxiety in the future, we're only beginning to understand all its implications as affective scientists work together to hammer out the details.[20] For now, let's turn to some established ways that mental health practitioners have used to diagnose and treat anxiety.

DIAGNOSIS

Even though anxiety is the most diagnosed mental health condition, I suspect that it is significantly *under*diagnosed. This is partially because lots of people still prefer not to talk about mental health, let alone pursue treatment. For every one of my patients who comes to see me about their anxiety, I'm sure there are many people struggling with similar issues who don't seek out help. But amid the challenging events of recent years, I've been heartened to see a more open dialogue about anxiety and other mental health issues. Entertainers, athletes, and other public figures have opened up about their own mental health challenges, and the stubborn stigmas around suffering from anxiety are starting to crumble.

When Should I Seek Care?

You know anxiety is serious when it disrupts your day-to-day ability to function in social situations and at work. In this book, we will meet a number of my former patients who got to a point where their anxiety was getting in the way of their friendships, their family relationships, their success at work, and even their ability to simply leave their homes and go out into the world. Ask yourself: if I were not anxious, would my social and work life be better? If the answer is yes, then finding a way to address your anxiety is important.

It can be easy to minimize your feelings of anxiety, telling yourself to toughen up or get over it — this often mirrors advice from others who may not understand your problems, or who may have neglected to look after their own mental health. But I assure you that opening up and getting help from a mental health professional will benefit you in the long run, and it might even save your life; serious anxiety may lead to an inability to care for yourself as well as suicidal or even homicidal thoughts. While most anxious people will never reach those extremes, it's best to start treatment before the problem feels urgent.

If you're not yet ready to seek out a mental health professional, mention your anxious feelings to your general practitioner. They will be able to advise you on your options for seeking further treatment, as well as test for other medical conditions that may be contributing to your anxiety.

Even when people do seek care, there are challenges with how anxiety is diagnosed. The current edition of the American Psychiatric Association's *Diagnostic and Statistical Manual of Mental Disorders*, or *DSM-5-TR*, breaks anxiety down into several disorders, such as generalized anxiety disorder (GAD), separation anxiety disorder, panic disorder, and specific phobias, each with a distinctive set of symptoms psychiatrists can use to make a quantifiable diagnosis. However, many clinicians, including myself, have found the *DSM*'s approach lacking, too inflexible to meet the needs of the complicated spectrum of human mental health. These specific disorders have their uses in clinical and research work—for instance, we will see many studies where research participants are diagnosed via these *DSM*-dictated criteria—but I don't believe they are adequate to capture the broad range of ways that anxiety can manifest in the modern world.

In other words, you don't have to have a textbook disorder to be hamstrung by anxiety. Even if your symptoms don't fall perfectly into any of the *DSM*'s categories, anxiety can be a real threat to your productivity and well-being. The COVID-19 pandemic, and being in lockdown, highlighted the importance of mental health, clarifying the concept that many people were suffering even if they didn't meet the formal diagnostic criteria for anxiety. Ill effects manifested as poor sleep (the "coronasomnia" that I suffered from during the early days of the pandemic), nausea, headaches, spiraling worries, or even just feeling "blah." Some self-medicated with an extra glass or two of wine or an extra scoop of ice cream at night, but many others sought out healthier solutions, and my hope is that some lasting good will come out of such a difficult period, as people retain strategies for coping with anxiety into the future.

My advice to patients and friends is to try not to get too hung up on the formal classifications and diagnoses of anxiety. As a psychiatrist, I have the utmost respect for mental health professionals who are performing research and treating patients clinically. But I'm also a realist, and I understand that not every person who struggles with anxiety is going to fit perfectly into the strictures of the *DSM*, whether from a unique profile of symptoms or simply from an inability to access professional care because of cost, time, or location. I urge you not to let that keep you from pursuing relief from anxiety through the healthy, zero-risk nutritional strategies I will discuss in this book.

WHAT ABOUT DEPRESSION?

Depression and anxiety are often mentioned together, and with good reason. Depression is the second most diagnosed mental health condition, and many patients experience both, either at different times or all at once. Evidence has shown that up to 85 percent of depressed patients also have significant anxiety, and 90 percent of patients with an anxiety disorder experience depression.[21] In my clinical experience, I can generally diagnose which of the two is causing a patient the most problems, but that doesn't mean the other is totally absent. The lines are not always as clear as we would like them to be, because of the complexity and unpredictability of the human brain.

Often, it's not essential to fully disambiguate depression from anxiety, because the treatments for both have a lot of overlap. For the purposes of this book, I've primarily focused on research into anxiety specifically, but I'll also incorporate a few particularly interesting studies that focus on both conditions or even focus primarily on depression, with an understanding that they are so tightly intertwined.

If you've experienced depression — either with or without anxiety — many of the recommendations in this book may very well help you, even if they're not explicitly depression focused. And if you're not sure which one you're struggling with, take heart that you're likely to improve both at once as you follow the suggestions here. This is why food is such a powerful, flexible tool to add to your mental fitness tool kit — eating healthy, whole foods is always going to help your physical and mental health in a variety of ways, no matter what your specific struggle. The power is at the end of your fork.

TREATMENTS FOR ANXIETY

There is a broad range of treatments for anxiety, and different patients find success through different methods. In our modern world, "treatment" tends to send our minds to pharmaceuticals, which are certainly one valuable tool. Drugs that seek to rebalance brain chemistry and increase levels of certain key neurotransmitters, like selective serotonin reuptake inhibitors (SSRIs) — which boost levels of the mood-modulating neurotransmitter serotonin — are often prescribed for long-term anxiety, and sedatives like benzodiazepines can be helpful for management of acute anxiety attacks. Anxiety drugs are being prescribed at record rates. During the early stages of the COVID-19 pandemic, prescriptions of the SSRI Zoloft (sertraline) increased more than 20 percent between February and March 2020, ultimately driving the drug into a worldwide shortage.[22] But while pharmaceuticals can be effective, there is no single wonder drug that works for everyone, and some people don't respond to them at all. Furthermore, drugs come with their own problems in the form of side effects and even dependencies. Though they can be an important piece of the puzzle, no one should expect a magical pill that fully cures anxiety, and they should only be taken under guidance from a doctor or psychiatrist.

Many anxiety sufferers also find relief through psychotherapy. One popular therapy for treating anxiety is cognitive behavioral therapy (CBT), which is a highly structured form aimed at changing the thinking patterns and beliefs that lead to anxiety. One technique in CBT is exposure therapy, which aims to intentionally expose the patient to anxiety-inducing situations to teach them to recognize when their brains are sending up false alarms about perceived threats. While CBT has been a longtime strategy for anxiety sufferers, studies on its effectiveness have been mixed.[23]

While psychotherapy doesn't come with side effects like anxiety drugs, its cost can put it outside the means of many people, and the time commitment can be difficult to fit into a busy schedule. Even for those resolved to seek treatment through therapy, it can be difficult to find an available provider, with shortages of therapists facing down an increased patient load. Even in major metropolitan areas, it can be tough to find a doctor who is taking patients, but in many rural areas there are simply no psychiatrists to be found. More than half of US counties don't have a psychiatrist, which means long travel and wait times. There are signs that the future may be brighter, due to increased numbers of psychiatry residents and young people who are in tune with the value of becoming a mental health practitioner.[24] But that doesn't help you if you need care now.

During the height of the COVID-19 pandemic, telehealth became a necessary tool for me and other mental health professionals to provide care. And even now that in-person appointments are possible again, telehealth remains a viable option that expands access to mental health care. While I prefer seeing patients in person, recent studies have shown that there aren't significant differences in results between in-person and remote care.[25] So, finding an online practitioner could be the right choice for you.

Beyond more formalized treatments, there are plenty of other ways to try to alleviate anxiety. After my cancer diagnosis, I found comfort in simply walking outside and breathing more mindfully. I was careful to reframe my thoughts to focus on the positives in the situation, and to avoid the news and other stimuli that I knew could send me into an anxious spiral. I also practiced Transcendental Meditation, which has been shown to help lower anxiety.[26] I revisited what my grandparents taught me about pranayama yoga — the breathing exercises that helped me before my meeting with the Prince of Wales.[27] I've had patients swear by exercise as a way to calm their minds, which has also been substantiated by research.[28] Even something as simple as staying hydrated by drinking water has been shown to make a difference.[29]

Anxiety can be reduced by discovering a new interest or passion. During my visit to London, I was introduced to a woman who had spent years warped by anxiety and a myriad of other mental conditions that kept her bedridden and medicated. Though there were a variety of factors in her recovery, the most important was her discovery of art through a free class she learned about from a pamphlet in a doctor's office. Creating art gave her a venue to express her deepest emotions, which helped her unwind from years of being tortured by anxiety. Today she lives a happy, healthy, anxiety-free life while helping others through her amazing work in mental health advocacy.

There are also a multitude of resources in print and online to help manage anxiety. Two books I recommend are *Feel the Fear...and Do It Anyway* by Dr. Susan Jeffers, and *Life Unlocked* by Dr. Srinivasan Pillay, both of which offer practical advice on how to deal with fear and anxiety. For apps, I like Calm (https://www.calm.com) and Headspace (https://www.headspace.com), which provide meditation solutions. Reulay (https://www.reulay.com), which I am on the board of advisers for, offers research-based solutions for anxiety. CIRCA (https://circa.world) is an app that offers brain-based solutions for anxiety.

Clearly, people around the world are embracing different ways to escape anxiety's clutches. In the APA's January 2022 Healthy Minds Monthly poll, one in four Americans reported making a mental health–related New Year's resolution, including plans to meditate, see a therapist or psychiatrist, detox from social media, start a journaling practice, and use a mental health app.[30] Every brain is different, and I've seen repeatedly in my clinic that different patients respond to diverse therapies.

While all of these are important strategies for easing anxiety and putting yourself on the right track to a healthy mind, there are still significant challenges to treating anxiety in an effective and lasting way. Most clinical trials of anxiety disorders document response rates of 50–60 percent and remission rates between 25 percent and 35 percent.[31] This means that up to 75 percent of people treated for anxiety may never get better. While that daunting statistic is certainly a testament to what a worthy adversary anxiety can be, it's also a sign that until recently, anxiety treatments haven't accounted for the fact that it's a condition of both mind *and* body. Consequently, treatment plans often leave out the most accessible and important tool to improve your mental health: your diet.

THE PROMISE OF NUTRITIONAL PSYCHIATRY

Being careful about the food you eat is certainly not a novel concept for health-conscious people in the twenty-first century. In parallel with the anxiety epidemic, the world is also suffering through an epidemic of bad health outcomes linked to poor diet. According to the World Health Organization, 650 million adults, 340 million adolescents, and 39 million children are obese.[32] That's more than 1 billion people! In the United States, the prevalence of obesity is over 40 percent and growing, with a corresponding rise in obesity-related conditions such as heart disease, stroke, and metabolic conditions including type 2 diabetes.[33] Whether your priority is maintaining a healthy weight, managing levels of cholesterol and blood sugar, or simply trying to eat ethically and sustainably in an era of climate change and factory farms, there is an avalanche of advice and eating plans out there.

But while connections between the food you eat and conditions like diabetes and heart disease have long been clear, science is just starting to catch up with the crucial truth that your diet and metabolic health also shape your mental health.

Not long ago, my trio of areas of study — nutrition, culinary arts, and psychiatry — might have seemed like an odd mashup of interests. But over the last decade or so, scientific research has led us to understand that these twin epidemics of mental and physical health are linked. As we'll see in later chapters, conditions like gut dysbiosis, chronic inflammation, and metabolic diseases are often implicated in causing anxiety. The opposite is true, too — in nearly all these conditions, anxiety has been shown to cause or worsen symptoms of physical health. The field of medical research that reveals the ways in which the food you eat affects your feelings and mood is called nutritional psychiatry.

In part 1 of this book, we are going to thoroughly explore the latest research concerning the connection between diet and anxiety, exploring the science behind why these associations exist and how the damage can be reversed. While this material may feel dense at times, that's a reflection of how many different body systems contribute to anxiety and the wealth of studies that have unpacked these associations over the past few years — and I promise that having a firm understanding of the science will make your anti-anxiety meals that much more delicious! In chapter 2, we'll learn the basics of the gut-brain connection and how the trillions of bacteria living in your gut are one of the most important factors in controlling anxiety. In chapter 3, we will delve into how the connections between your gut and your mental health also involve your immune system, due to the high concentration of immune processes in your gut mucosa. In chapter 4, we'll cover how poor diet choices can contribute to chronic inflammation in your body and brain that can exacerbate anxiety. In chapter 5 we'll learn how a compound called leptin controls your appetite and shapes your response to anxiety. In chapter 6, we'll explore the links between metabolism and mental health, establishing how anxiety can be both a byproduct and a cause of the metabolic disorders that represent one of the most serious threats to health in the modern world.

Once we've built a firm understanding of the different processes through which diet affects anxiety, we'll learn how to establish eating habits that ensure that your body has the right tools to master your anxiety. In part 2, we'll learn about different macronutrients, micronutrients, and bioactives and phytochemicals that can help alleviate anxiety, and develop brain-healthy food-buying habits, while also helping you avoid foods that can leave you vulnerable. And in part 3, we'll take that knowledge and examine how to build an eating plan that will help you prioritize anxiety-fighting foods. Finally, I've designed a set of recipes based on my training as a professional chef and my experience with patients in my clinic, giving you ways to create delicious antianxiety meals that will fit into your busy life.

As we navigate the connections between diet and anxiety, we'll be on the cutting edge of research of some of the most exciting frontiers in medical science. But what I want you to remember above all is that by calming your mind with food, you are harnessing the power of one of the most fundamental parts of human life. You *must* eat to survive; there's no getting around that simple fact. So I encourage you to give careful consideration to your dietary choices, building your lifestyle around healthy whole foods full of the right balance of macro- and micronutrients that will keep you thriving in both body and mind.

To start, let's learn the basics of the most important interplay between your brain and body: the connection between your brain and your gut.

CHAPTER TWO

Gut Feelings

In the fourth century BC, Hippocrates, the father of modern medicine, shared a prescient opinion that "bad digestion is the root of all evil," and that "death sits in the bowels."[1]

In the seventeenth century, Dutch scientist Antoni van Leeuwenhoek used homemade single-lens microscopes on samples gathered from his own body to make the first observations of bacteria. Describing his remarkable discovery, he said, "I then most always saw, with great wonder, that in the said matter there were many very little living animalcules, very prettily a-moving."[2]

In the nineteenth century, French zoologist Élie Metchnikoff believed that bacteria in fermented milk were beneficial in fighting "autointoxication," a term used to describe a wide range of symptoms from fatigue to melancholia. His theory that eating yogurt could delay senility and enhance health was popular during his time but soon faded from prominence for more than a century.[3]

Starting in the late twentieth century and continuing through today, modern medical research has begun to knit together these foundational ideas, creating a full understanding of the incredible influence of tiny bacteria on an organism as large and complex as a human being. Hippocrates was correct about how much influence the digestive tract has on the rest of the body—though I suspect even he would be surprised by how profoundly our guts shape how we think and feel. Van Leeuwenhoek helped us understand both the threat and usefulness of the microscopic organisms that colonize our bodies. Metchnikoff's theory about yogurt became the basis of modern probiotic use, establishing the idea that eating food that encourages bacterial growth can improve gut health.

Finally, in 2001, Nobel laureate Joshua Lederberg first used the term "microbiome" to refer to the vast array of microorganisms that live in your body.[4] Over the following decades, medical researchers have proven that a healthy brain relies on a healthy gut, and a healthy gut relies on fostering a healthy microbiome, creating a foundational pillar of nutritional psychiatry and opening up a new way of thinking about mental health.

To understand these ideas more fully, let's examine the different connections between the gut and the brain and then take a closer look at the influence of the microbiome.

CONNECTIONS BETWEEN THE GUT AND THE BRAIN

Plato famously described reason and emotion as two horses pulling us in opposite directions, creating the conception of human judgment as a tug-of-war between our rational "head," and our passionate "heart." This dichotomy was further developed by Enlightenment thinkers like Thomas Jefferson, who wrote a dialogue between his head and his heart in a 1786 love letter,[5] and the concept of a warring head and heart is still commonly referenced today. Alongside our heads and hearts, there's another part of the body that's associated with thoughts and feelings: our guts. In common usage, our guts are the root of our being, the nexus of everything we just *know*. When you show bravery and resolve, you "have guts." When you act on a hunch, you "trust your gut." When you really detest someone, you "hate their guts." Clearly, we have an innate understanding of the importance of the gut in developing and expressing emotions — even if the medical establishment hasn't, until recently, understood the gut as a fulcrum of mental health.

Of course, with a more refined and literal understanding of physiology, we can see the practical limits of these metaphors. We know that our brains process the whole range of emotions, not just cold, calculating rational thought. Our hearts are far too busy pumping blood to truly be the anatomical center of emotion and desire. And our guts don't have a special power to strengthen our resolve or put together the pieces of a mystery. Still, modern research has proven that our guts *do* play an essential role in regulating our emotions, and disruptions in the gut can lead to mental struggles — including anxiety.

Over the years in my clinic, I've found that it can be hard for my patients to internalize the gut's role in mental health. I agree that it's counterintuitive that two such physically distant organ systems would be so tightly tied together. I also suspect there's an element of disbelief that the humble guts, tasked with the mucky process of separating nutrients from waste, could influence something as lofty as the mind's ability to process the world around us. I want to dispel this conception of the gut as a grimy fuel refinery and reimagine it as a bustling city whose residents — a host of helpful bacteria — perform essential work to keep the digestive, immune, and nervous systems operating smoothly.

It's important to remember that your gut and brain weren't always two distinct organ systems. Whether in the womb or in a test tube, you start as a zygote, or fertilized egg, which is formed when a sperm and egg unite. From that zygote, trillions of little cells grow and develop to form the parts of your body, from the largest organ, your skin, to the tiniest structures within your beautiful brain. Your central nervous system (CNS), made up of your brain and spinal cord, is formed by special cells known as neural crest cells. These cells migrate throughout the developing embryo, especially to what will become your gut, forming what we call the enteric nervous system (ENS), a network of nerves that control gastrointestinal operations. The ENS contains between 100 and 500 million neurons, the largest collection of nerve cells in the body — larger even than the brain. That's why some experts call the gut "the second brain."

The ENS is considered part of the ANS, which plays an important role in stress response and controls an array of involuntary bodily processes, like your heartbeat, breathing, and pupil dilation. The ENS, separate from the CNS, can operate without any direct input from your brain. But just because the two are independent doesn't mean they don't communicate. In fact, they stay in close touch, sending messages back and forth in a near-constant cross talk, like teenagers glued to their phones, texting each other about every tiny development of the day.

The major conduit for these messages is the vagus nerve — often called the "wanderer nerve" because of the winding distance it travels in your body. The vagus nerve connects your brain stem to your gut wall, creating a physical link between your digestive tract and your CNS. With assistance from connections through a set of smaller nerves called the spinal sensory nerves, the vagus nerve provides a pathway for nerve impulses to travel back and forth, carrying crucial messages. Hormones, neurotransmitters, inflammatory markers, and immune signals can also travel between the gut and brain via the circulatory system, providing other pathways for communication and collaboration.[6]

Why do the gut and brain need to talk? Much of the communication is about monitoring digestion, regulating appetite, keeping tabs on ingested food, and breaking food down for fuel. But the gut and brain also communicate about mood. You're probably familiar with the uncomfortable rumble of nervous indigestion during stressful times, or the unsettling feeling of "butterflies in your stomach" when you feel nervous or excited. Both are examples of how the gut and brain communicate along the vagus nerve, keeping the CNS and the digestive tract on the same page.

A bit of nervous indigestion is no cause for concern, but there are also clear links between mental health problems and more serious digestive issues. For example, the gastrointestinal disorder irritable bowel syndrome (IBS) is often linked with disorders like anxiety and depression. You might think that IBS would be a root cause of anxiety due to the constant fear of your bowels acting up in a place where you don't have easy access to a restroom. But, in fact, scientists have observed the opposite effect: anxiety can be the root cause of IBS, and IBS can be treated with interventions aimed at mental health, like psychotherapy and SSRIs.[7] Anxiety has also been implicated in causing or worsening other serious digestive conditions, such as acid reflux[8] and peptic ulcers.[9]

Clearly your gut and brain are deeply intertwined physiologically, each helping the other perform the vital tasks necessary to keep you happy and healthy. But as I've already hinted, there is a third major player in their dynamic. To further understand the relationship between the gut and the brain, it's essential to learn more about the role of your gut microbiome.

THE GUT MICROBIOME

The most important participant in the gut-brain connection isn't actually part of *you* at all; it's another organism entirely. Or more accurately, it's *trillions* of other organisms: the bacteria that make up your gut microbiome along with their genetic material. We are superorganisms made up of our human cells as well as the cells of our microbiome, and we need both systems to be working in harmonious symbiosis for us to survive. To paraphrase Walt Whitman's "Song of Myself," you *do* contain multitudes — of bacteria.

It's worth noting that your microbiome isn't limited to just your digestive tract, nor is it made up solely of bacteria. Your microbiome also includes viruses, fungi, protozoa, and archaea that live in your gut, but also on your skin and in your mouth, nasal passages, and urogenital tract. All over your body, these microorganisms play a role in important bodily functions. Your microbiota outnumber your own human cells 10 to 1, and they can be made up of more than a thousand different species.[10] They contain anywhere from 2 million to 20 million genes, while the human genome contains an estimated twenty thousand to twenty-five thousand genes. In other words, the microbiome can represent up to 99.9 percent of the genetic material present in the human body.[11] When you retool your perspective to take into account the sheer number and variety of microbiota living in your body, it would be hard to believe that they *didn't* have a huge influence on your health.

At the beginning of this chapter, we saw a few glimpses of the scientific history that helped us reach an understanding of the microbiome's importance, as scientists and thinkers studied the gut's role in health and bacteria's role throughout the natural world. But following Joshua Lederberg's initial use of the term "microbiome" in 2001, research on the role of the microbiome in the human body has exploded. In 2007, the National Institutes of Health launched the Human Microbiome Project.[12] The major goal of the first phase of this project was to characterize the genomic makeup of all microbes living in the human body. Once scientists understood what microbes were present, in 2014, the Human Microbiome Project moved into its second phase, which focused on understanding their functioning and actions.

Thanks to the Human Microbiome Project — and similar projects in the United Kingdom and Europe — we are developing a strong understanding of the various roles the gut microbiome takes on. Among many other tasks, gut microbiota help us break down nutrients in food, produce vitamins and other nutrients, modulate the nervous system and hormone responses, and support detoxification in the body. They can control our response to certain medications, and they influence and train our immune system, help-ing to fight dangerous pathogens (we'll expand on the microbiome's role in the immune system in chapter 3). Disruptions in the gut microbiome have been linked to a vast array of medical conditions, from IBS, which we've already discussed, to asthma, skin conditions like eczema, arthritis, type 2 diabetes, cardiovascular disease, auto-immune conditions, and even Alzheimer's disease.[13] Most important for our purposes, gut microbiota play a crucial role in mental health, ensuring a proper supply of the chemicals that can ward off condi-tions like anxiety.

The Malleable Microbiome

Given the importance of the microbiome, you might think that the makeup of bacteria in the body is carefully planned and finely cali-brated in an exact recipe for perfect health. Unfortunately, it's not that simple. The makeup and balance of different species in the gut microbiome are astonishingly unique to each individual; while any two people share 99.9 percent of their own human genome, they could have up to a 90 percent *difference* in the composition of their gut microbiome.[14] That means that the microbiome is heavily indi-vidualized, much like our thumbprints, and what is healthy and balanced in one person might look totally different in another.

Furthermore, the makeup of your microbiome is not static. It's constantly responding and changing, a process that scientists call "microbial succession." Some of these changes happen on a short timescale, like how your microbiome shifts with your body's circa-dian rhythm, or internal clock, as you move from day into night. Other changes happen across your whole lifetime, with different microbial patterns evident from birth into childhood into adult-hood into old age. Environmental factors can also change your microbiome. For instance, a course of antibiotics can wreak havoc on certain strains of bacteria, leaving others to flourish, causing disruptions in your gut. Such an imbalance in the composition of your gut bacteria is called gut dysbiosis, and we'll see many ways that it can lead to poor health outcomes.

The most significant environmental factor for maintaining a healthy gut microbiome — and the one over which you have the greatest control — is your diet. The food you eat has a major influence on the balance of your microbiota, because your diet is also your microbiome's diet. You've heard that pregnant mothers are "eating for two," but really every person in the world is always eating for *trillions*. And since different types of bacteria thrive on different kinds of nutrients, changes in food supply can lead to vast swings in bacterial populations. It's crucial to feed your microbiome in a way that promotes helpful bacteria and discourages harmful ones.

For an illustration of how your diet shapes your gut microbiome, consider the people of the Hadza tribe of Tanzania, who were the subject of a landmark study by a group of Stanford microbiology researchers.[15] The Hadza are hunter-gatherers, and they eat a very different diet in the wet season than in the dry season. By monitoring Hadza stool samples over the course of a year, the researchers found that the makeup of their microbiomes fluctuated as their diets changed. In the wet season, when their diet was rich in honey and berries, their microbiomes were robust and diverse. In the dry season, when they ate more meat and had less variety in their diet, their microbiomes showed less diversity. When the wet season rolled around again, their microbiomes recovered to their previous state.

The lesson of the Hadza is important even for those of us who don't follow a seasonal hunter-gatherer diet. When you take care of your gut microbiome, it takes care of you. Eating foods that promote healthy bacterial growth is crucial for your well-being, but a poor diet can throw everything off. We'll go into more detail about the individual foods and overall diets that promote gut health in parts 2 and 3, but for now, the important point is to understand that maintaining a healthy gut microbiome takes work. I encourage you to think of your microbiota as something you need to take care of every day, just like brushing your teeth or taking a shower. That might mean eating probiotic foods like plain yogurt, which contain live, healthy bacteria that reinforce your existing gut microbiome; eating prebiotic foods like onions, leeks, and garlic, which give your good bacteria food to eat; or simply avoiding foods like sugar, which allow your bad bacteria to thrive. Making microbiome maintenance part of your daily routine is important to your mental well-being. This has been such an important factor in the health of my clients. I love it when they connect these dots and start to adapt their eating behaviors to promote a healthy gut.

A Bidirectional Relationship

The two-way communication between the gut and the brain means that trouble in either location can reverberate in the other. Just as an unhealthy diet can throw your gut microbiome off balance and drag down your mental health, mental stresses like anxiety can also cause disruptions in your microbiome. Much of the research around how your mood can disrupt your gut comes from the studies on IBS—clear links have been established to show that people suffering from anxiety and depression are more likely to develop IBS. But you don't need to develop IBS to suffer from disruption in your microbiome. Studies have shown that even a two-hour exposure to stressful situations can cause significant alterations in bacterial communities and proportions in the gut.[16]

In a healthy gut and brain, a properly balanced microbiome leads to good mental health, which in turn further reinforces the microbiome. But with an unhealthy diet and an anxious brain, an imbalanced microbiome leads to further trouble in the brain, which can then knock your microbiome out of whack. The nature of this bidirectional relationship often leads my patients to feel daunted and overwhelmed, unsure of where the cycle of eating and mental health begins and ends. But instead of giving up with your head spinning, I encourage you to think of this as liberating.

Understanding how to eat for your mental health, especially when suffering from anxiety, is like always having the right answer on a test: no matter where the issue is rooted, the solution is always to eat a diet rich in brain-healthy foods, like berries, salmon, and olive oil.

To further understand how disruptions in the gut microbiome can worsen anxiety, let's meet a former patient of mine who found that misguided dietary changes led to an increase in anxious feelings.

THE ANXIOUS GUT

Tilo was a middle-aged woman who had spent much of her life struggling with her weight. A year or so before she came to see me, she joined a group weight-loss program at work and found that the support of her friends and coworkers helped her start slimming down. She lost close to 20 pounds relatively quickly, which made her feel better emotionally and physically. Stubborn back and knee pain resolved with the weight loss, meaning she seldom needed the over-the-counter medication she'd been taking to help with those aches. For at least a little while, she was feeling great.

Unfortunately, after the initial burst of positivity surrounding her weight loss, she began feeling anxious. When she first came to see me in hope of turning around her mental health, she felt her anxiety was related to a plateau in her weight loss. After the first 20 pounds, she had difficulty losing the last 5 to reach her goal weight, and she was frustrated by the lack of success. She woke up every morning with a new feeling of dread, her heart racing as she worried about how she'd get through her day without checking the scale and agonizing over the pounds she could not shed. At first, she thought her anxiety-driven snacking was preventing her from losing weight, but she was quite diligent about tracking her food. As she drove to work, she would review in her head the foods she was carrying in her lunch bag to make certain she would not be overeating or miscounting calories.

As I got to know Tilo, I began to understand that she'd had mild anxiety prior to her weight-loss journey but was able to manage it by taking Zumba and hip-hop dance classes, which helped her "shake off" the feeling. But now she felt restless and was sleeping poorly, and her usual strategies weren't enough to get her anxiety under control.

As we discussed her dietary history, I could tell she had a particular issue with sugar. She recognized that high sugar intake was a problem and had worked very hard to cut back, using the weight-loss program's calorie-counting system. She was consuming the recommended number of calories for the day and paying attention to her micro- and macronutrients. But when I looked over her eating plan, I saw that she was still consuming refined sugar in various treats that were approved by the program since their low-calorie content meshed with the diet program's point-system requirement. Some were sweetened with things like agave nectar and beet syrup — sweeteners that might sound wholesome and pure, but sugar by any other name is still sugar! On food labels, you'll see more than 260 names for sugar, but your body doesn't differentiate based on marketing tactics.[17] The treats recommended by the diet plan were sweetened with low-calorie sweeteners like sucralose (sold under the brand name Splenda) — but unfortunately these are also known to leave you prone to gut dysbiosis.

I encouraged her to stop eating all the sources of sugar and artificial sweeteners for a full week, regardless of whether they were approved by her diet plan. While this was hard for her, she ate small servings of blueberries and plain probiotic-rich yogurt mixed with cinnamon and nut butter to help her sweet tooth along and avoid sugar-withdrawal symptoms. Over time we gradually added small servings of an "ice cream" made from fruit, but we continued to replace refined sugars in her food, even switching out her ketchup and salad dressing. She started to drink plain water flavored with citrus instead of the program-approved flavored low-calorie drink mix, which contained artificial sweeteners.

Tilo's anxiety started to subside within the first week of these nutritional changes, and over the following weeks the needle on the scale began to move again as well. She told me that it was like I had prescribed an anxiety medication, but all I did was teach her to be aware of how her diet choices were worsening her anxiety and give her some ways to satisfy her sweet tooth without wrecking her mental health.

If you're guessing that Tilo's problem was rooted in her gut, you're correct. But what exactly was going on? If her diet was sugar-heavy before she went on the weight-loss program, why would her anxiety worsen when she *cut down* on sugar, even if she didn't totally eliminate it? The answer is complicated, but it has to do with changes in her gut microbiome.

Many studies have confirmed links between sugar intake and anxiety,[18] and sugar is also a major culprit in microbiome disruption, creating an environment where good bacteria are prone to being choked out by bad bacteria. I suspect that accounts for Tilo's mild anxiety from before her weight-loss program, which she was able to manage through her exercise routine. But when she made dietary changes, replacing much of the sugar with low-calorie substitutes, her gut microbiome shifted further. The reason low-calorie sweeteners like sucralose can taste sweet without adding calories is that your gut can't absorb the sugars they contain. Your taste buds register sweetness, but the rest of your body does not, giving you a way to satisfy your sweet tooth without packing on pounds. But just because *you* can't process these types of sugars doesn't mean that your gut microbiota can't. Just as a horse can subsist on eating grass that our bodies cannot process, some bacteria can thrive on a diet of sweeteners that our bodies simply pass through. If those sugars aren't being absorbed by your large and small intestines, that means they are even more available for gut bacteria to feast on.[19] In Tilo's case, that meant an overgrowth of bad bacteria that took its toll in the form of heightened anxiety, which had to be corrected by limiting sugar *and* sweeteners.

Tilo's experience is a good reminder that losing weight and being healthy aren't necessarily the same thing. While it was great for her to drop weight she'd long struggled to lose, doing it through unhealthy diet practices led to disruptions in her gut microbiome and consequently increased anxiety. By moving her to a diet based on whole foods and low sugar intake without artificial sweeteners, we were able to help her lose more weight while also repairing the damage to her mental health and ensuring that her gut had the right tools to keep her anxiety-free.

THE NEUROTRANSMITTER FACTORY

By now we have a firm understanding that the gut microbiome plays a key role in anxiety. But *why* is this the case? What do gut microbiota actually *do* that creates changes in your brain?

One of the crucial roles of your gut microbiome is to help your body produce neurotransmitters, chemicals that carry messages between your nerve cells. Neurotransmitters are essential to a wide range of bodily functions — including movement and organ processes, like keeping your heart beating — but they are particularly notable for their role in cognition and mood. Neurotransmitters like serotonin, dopamine, and gamma-aminobutyric acid (GABA) are all important in regulating brain function, and imbalances in neurotransmitter levels are a key factor in a range of mental health disorders including depression and anxiety.

Your gut bacteria have a key role in producing these neurotransmitters. As gut bacteria break down, or metabolize, their food, they create substances called metabolites, which influence neurotransmitter production. Many of these metabolites are neurotransmitter precursors, building blocks that your body can assemble into complete neurotransmitter molecules. Others help trigger your body to make more neurotransmitters and to know when to release them.

Much of this neurotransmitter synthesis happens locally in the gut, where neurotransmitters help the ENS regulate processes of digestion. The most important neurotransmitters, however, are the ones in your brain; that's where an upset in the chemical balance can cause anxiety. Keeping your brain stocked with neurotransmitters isn't quite as simple as building them in your gut and shipping them up to your brain. As a protective measure, your body keeps your brain sealed off from your bloodstream through a complex defense system called the blood-brain barrier.[20] Neurotransmitters cannot cross the blood-brain barrier, but their precursors can. So, precursors made by your gut bacteria are carried through your bloodstream, across the blood-brain barrier, and into the brain, where they are assembled into the neurotransmitters that help control your emotions.[21]

Consider serotonin. Serotonin is an inhibitory neurotransmitter, which means it helps calm down your nerve cells, soothing them out of a frenzied state. Serotonin is thought to be one of the most crucial brain chemicals when it comes to anxiety; the most common type of drug prescribed to fight anxiety and depression is the SSRI, which increases levels of serotonin in the brain. While serotonin plays a key role in your mood and emotions, 95 percent of your body's serotonin is produced in the gut, most of which stays in your digestive tract to help the ENS regulate digestion.[22] Only 1–2 percent of your body's serotonin is produced in the brain.

Serotonin's precursor is the amino acid tryptophan, which you obtain through dietary sources like poultry and chickpeas (we'll cover more sources of tryptophan in chapter 7). Your body relies on gut bacteria to metabolize tryptophan from the food you eat, creating a variety of metabolites and signaling a vast, complicated set of processes that lead to serotonin synthesis in both the gut and the brain. Every step of the process is influenced by a variety of different strains of gut bacteria.[23]

Take a moment to absorb that. Healthy brain function requires the right amount of serotonin. Making enough serotonin relies on both eating the right nutrients and having the right bacteria in your gut to facilitate the process of turning those nutrients into serotonin. Therefore, if either of these factors breaks down — either you don't get enough dietary tryptophan or you don't have a well-balanced gut microbiome — your brain could run short of serotonin. And running short of serotonin puts you at risk for anxiety.

Taking an SSRI could very well help straighten out your serotonin levels, but SSRIs can have side effects and often require an arduous process of finding the right combination of drug and dosage. On the other hand, changing your diet to promote gut health and give you a steady supply of dietary tryptophan is a no-risk first step that can achieve the same end goal as pharmaceuticals. While medication is certainly useful and even necessary in many cases, I feel strongly that dietary interventions are the right place to start. But they are often overlooked.

I want to be clear that serotonin is not the entire picture, but just one of many compounds that play a role in mental health. In fact, in 2022, a much-discussed study posited that serotonin is not as important in depression and anxiety as has long been accepted.[24] But while that uncertainty can feel frustrating to those seeking to understand their mental health, I feel that it provides another strong argument for practicing nutritional psychiatry. Good gut health and nutrition don't just boost serotonin production; they also help ensure proper levels of a variety of other neurotransmitters, all of which play a role in your mental well-being.

For example, the neurotransmitter GABA is another central player in modulating anxiety response, particularly in the amygdala — the part of the brain described in chapter 1 as the flashpoint for anxiety. GABA is also an inhibitory neurotransmitter, and when GABA levels are low, your amygdala can be more reactive, triggering strong stress responses when they're not warranted. Your brain is missing an important tool for keeping extreme moods under control, which can contribute significantly to anxiety. GABA has been shown to be produced by certain gut bacteria, including *Bifidobacterium adolescentis*, so a gut imbalance that leads to a shortage of that species may mean a shortage of GABA in the gut and brain, thereby heightening the risk of anxiety.[25]

The same is true of the neurotransmitters dopamine, acetylcholine, and glutamate, among possibly others. Furthermore, neurotransmitters and their precursors aren't the only compounds made by gut bacteria that play an important role in the brain. Other compounds, like short-chain fatty acids (SCFAs) and brain-derived neurotrophic factor (BDNF), also have key roles in the relationship between gut and brain, and also rely on gut bacteria to create them.[26] BDNF assists with the stress response in the hippocampus and has been shown to fluctuate as gut microbiota change.[27] SCFAs are created by bacteria breaking down dietary fiber. Recent studies have shown that low levels of SCFAs can yield greater anxiety and depression, while higher levels can lead to a reduction in both conditions. Though most of this research is from preliminary animal studies, there is exciting potential in studying SCFAs more fully.[28]

TRUST YOUR GUT

Given the connections between anxiety and your gut, it's unsurprising that in a review of studies looking into the effectiveness of treating anxiety via the gut microbiome, the majority showed that participants' anxiety symptoms improved as their microbiomes became healthier. And in studies that showed positive results, the rate of efficacy of reducing anxiety was 86 percent—an extremely heartening number for a condition that is so notoriously difficult to treat. It's also important to note that studies where a probiotic supplement — a pill intended to foster bacterial growth in the gut — was used showed less reduction in anxiety than studies that relied on dietary changes.[29] That is another good sign that the most powerful medicine for combatting anxiety is a diet full of gut-healthy foods, such as probiotic-fermented foods like pickles and kimchi; prebiotics like garlic, onions, and bananas; and fiber-rich vegetables and whole grains.

And remember, if you are feeling like you don't quite understand the intricacies of the gut-brain connection, reassure yourself that even the world's leading experts don't understand all the details. What we *do* understand is that your gut bacteria know the secrets of a calm mind. By giving them the nourishment they need, you are trusting them to work on your behalf, laying the groundwork for good mental health and a life free of anxiety.

Gut dysbiosis is the most fundamental threat to mental health, and we will see how it is connected to all the other contributors to anxiety that we're going to discuss in the next few chapters. To start, let's turn to how a healthy gut and brain are essential to maintaining a healthy immune system.

CHAPTER THREE

Immune to Anxiety

Mary came to see me because her anxiety was out of control. At thirty-five years old, she and her husband decided it was finally time to have a baby, but it just wasn't happening. Difficulty getting pregnant was creating tension in her marriage, which left her either unable to go to sleep or waking up in the middle of the night feeling shaky and afraid. It had gotten so bad that, during the day, she was struggling to concentrate on tasks at work and at home.

Mary is not alone. Like many women her age, she was feeling the tension of having a full-time job and the pressure to have a family. Add in the stresses of a global pandemic and a host of other day-to-day fears, responsibilities, and frustrations, and it was easy to see how her anxiety could result from the accumulation of stresses in her life. But upon further examination, I noticed that something else might be at play.

As we spoke, I saw that she had a rash on both sides of her face, extending over both of her cheekbones in the shape of a butterfly's wing. She thought she might be reacting to a new face cream and told me she'd booked a dermatology appointment, but I suspected something more serious. The clinical name for this rash pattern is a "butterfly rash," and it is a telltale sign that a patient's immune system is attacking their own tissues. A leading culprit, especially in women of childbearing age, is an autoimmune disease called systemic lupus erythematosus, commonly known as lupus. Patients afflicted with this condition may have inflammation of several organ systems: the kidneys, skin, joints, blood, and nervous system can all be affected.[1] Although we don't fully understand how or why lupus develops in individual cases, we do understand that many of these organ changes are caused by an immune response in overdrive. Recent research has shown that the composition of our gut bacteria can be a major factor in lupus patients.[2] Stress and anxiety can disrupt the intestinal barrier, such that communication between the gut and brain breaks down. It's the biological equivalent of spotty cell service, leading to dropped calls and texts that won't go through as your communication falters. When this becomes chronic, a kind of metabolic confusion arises, which can contribute to the sort of abnormal immunity that can lead to conditions like lupus.[3]

Treating a complex disease like lupus is never an easy task. It's a condition with no true cure, but through a variety of treatments and therapies, most patients can bring their symptoms under control. I referred Mary to a primary care physician who worked closely with a rheumatologist and put her on a course of steroids to reduce her inflammation. I prescribed her an initial course of an SSRI and a benzodiazepine, traditional treatments for anxiety. But I also had a conversation with her about making major changes to her diet to comprehensively address her anxiety. We took an inventory of the less-than-healthy habits she had picked up over the pandemic. She admitted she had developed a passion for bubble tea—delicious but full of sugar—which I encouraged her to replace with a healthier Matcha Green "Bubble" Tea (see page 268). I coached her on how to add a higher dose of anti-inflammatory foods to her diet, which would bring back biodiversity to her gut microbiome: different colors, textures, sizes, and shapes of vegetables such as peppers, zucchini, summer squash, Brussels sprouts, cauliflower, beets, and more. I recommended she replace her inflammation-producing vegetable oil with olive oil, increase her consumption of fermented foods like miso and kimchi, amp up her omega-3s by adding wild sockeye salmon and anchovies, and opt for hemp milk instead of dairy milk (see page 267 for my Homemade Hemp Milk recipe). I will explain these specific recommendations later in the book, but the overall goal was to move her toward healthy whole foods and away from processed ingredients.

Mary had a good short-term response to the steroids, and the psychiatric medications helped somewhat, but when she came in for a follow-up visit, she was still struggling with both anxiety and her lupus symptoms. I asked her about the dietary changes, and she admitted that things had felt too hectic for her to change the way she ate in the middle of everything else going on in her life. I sympathized completely but encouraged her to start small and stay consistent, and I met with her and her husband to plan out meals, like Masala Baked Salmon (see page 244) and my Go-To Calm Green Salad (see page 255). She could prepare these ahead and use them on multiple days, making meal prep and planning easier.

Sure enough, once she committed to the dietary changes, we truly started to see shifts in her mood. Within just a month of consistently embracing an eating plan that was healthier for her gut and brain, she was feeling calmer and sleeping better. And as her anxiety waned, her lupus symptoms became easier to manage—a clear sign that her immune system function was improving. Mary couldn't believe that her diet was playing such a central role in both her mental health and her autoimmune disease, but I explained that until recently, no one—from patients like her all the way to the highest echelons of medicine—knew about the vital interplay between our gut bacteria, the immune system, and anxiety.

WAIT – WHAT'S CAUSING WHAT?

What was really going on inside Mary's body when she first came to see me? There were three major factors at play: her anxiety, which was centered in her brain; her gut microbiome, which was influenced by her diet; and her struggles with lupus, the result of disruptions in her immune system. It's tempting to try to determine a root cause and connect her issues together in a defined sequence of events. For instance, we might theorize that her anxiety arose first, which then led to disruptions in her gut and eventually her immune system. Or we might suspect that her imbalanced gut microbiome led to her anxiety, which set off her immune issues. Or maybe her immune issues arose first, which in turn altered her gut microbiota, triggering her anxiety.

Truthfully, *all* of these scenarios are possible. There are no one-way streets here. These three body systems are interconnected in a delicately balanced ecosystem, and the variety and breadth of their interactions are mind-boggling. But, as we've touched on before, it's important to realize that the primary cause *does not matter.* A disruption in any of these three systems is likely to lead to problems with the other two. Regardless of where the problem is rooted, the surest, most accessible, and easiest to control variable is the food you eat. As we saw with Mary, it wasn't enough to treat just the anxiety or the lupus; it was also crucial to treat her gut microbiome through changes in her diet. Only by taking care of all three systems was she able to get her total health back on track.

Since we have already explored the gut-brain connection, let's meet the immune system and learn about the mechanisms through which it influences your mental and digestive health—and vice versa.

WHAT IS IMMUNITY?

It's a dangerous world out there. Every living thing is constantly beset by a host of dangerous foreign invaders called pathogens. All organisms need defense mechanisms to protect against pathogens—or else they won't be living for long.[4]

I'm sure you're familiar with at least some of the work your immune system does. Everyone has been grateful for a "strong" immune system when that tickle in your throat fails to materialize into a cold or has lamented a "weak" immune system when you've gotten sick multiple times back-to-back. And during the rise of the COVID-19 pandemic, we all got a crash course in immunology from both a biological and epidemiological perspective, with talk of herd immunity, vaccine efficacy, and monoclonal antibodies. But despite knowing how important the immune system is, its actual mechanics can feel abstract and opaque. I want to demystify them here so that we're well prepared to learn about how immunity interacts with the gut and brain.

The immune system keeps every part of your body under constant surveillance, which requires a nimble and flexible approach. It needs to be active in your skin, your respiratory passages, your intestinal tract, and anywhere else pathogens, cancer cells, and toxins might appear. Many of the organs important to immunity are part of the lymphatic system — for instance, your bone marrow, where key immune cells are made; your lymph nodes; and your thymus. But the immune system's action isn't limited to one organ system. Your skin, mucous membranes, and (you guessed it!) gut are also crucial.

There are two different types of immunity: innate immunity and adaptive immunity. They operate in complementary but different ways, stepping in to protect your body from different kinds of pathogens and utilizing different sets of chemicals and antibodies to do their work. Both are essential to your body's ability to keep itself healthy.[5] Though the immune system's functions are complex enough to fill an entire book of their own, here's a brief overview of how these two types of immunity work to protect you.

Innate Immunity

Innate immunity is your body's first-line response to a foreign invader. It's like the body's paramedic team. When there is trouble, the innate immune system is ready to detect the problem and show up quickly on the scene with a trauma kit designed to handle emergencies. For instance, when you cut your finger, it is your innate immune system that rushes in to try to ensure that stray bacteria aren't allowed to blossom into a full-blown infection. Speed is essential, given how quickly some pathogens can grow into a real threat. And since your body has no way of knowing what foreign invaders will try to intrude, the innate immune system must be prepared to thwart pathogens it has never seen before.

The innate immune system locates trouble by zeroing in on certain warning signs. Researchers call these warning signs pathogen-associated molecular patterns. Once trouble is detected, immune cells produce cytokines, small proteins that are crucial to your immune cells' communication.[6] Cytokines act as the paramedic team's walkie-talkies, calling in reinforcements and making sure every responder is on the same page, part of a cohesive strategy to fight off the invaders.

Once trouble is detected and the right team has been assembled, the innate immune system can pull all kinds of different levers to slow down pathogens. It can create a more hostile environment for pathogens by altering the body's pH or raising its temperature (which you may experience as a fever). It can recruit a variety of leukocytes, or white blood cells, which perform many different functions to destroy pathogens. For example, phagocytes like macrophages and neutrophils specialize in gobbling up pathogens, engulfing and destroying them. Natural killer cells are named for their innate toxicity to certain viruses and tumor cells.[7] One of the main ways your immune system fights pathogens is by triggering inflammation, which brings leukocyte-rich blood to the problem area. As we saw with Mary at the beginning of the chapter, inflammation can be harmful as well as helpful — we will cover this in more detail in chapter 4.

The innate immune system uses a wealth of resources and

strategies to act as a first line of defense against pathogens. But there is a trade-off: innate immunity does not have "memory." While it is prepared to fight off pathogens your body has never seen before, it doesn't "learn" anything from the experience. The next time your innate immune system sees that same pathogen, it will trigger the same response, whether or not it was effective the first time. Some pathogens are sophisticated enough to overwhelm the paramedics, and longer-term help is needed. Luckily, they can get on their cytokine walkie-talkies and call for reinforcements.

Adaptive Immunity

If the innate immune system is your body's paramedic team, the adaptive immune system is an experienced group of medical researchers. They may not specialize in stopping bleeding or setting broken bones, but they excel at studying a disease inside and out, gradually building a body of knowledge to fight it more effectively and intelligently. While the innate immune system works from a standard tool set for different types of pathogens, the adaptive immune system builds a unique response for each pathogen and hones its approach with time and experience.

Adaptive immunity is called into action against a host of familiar infectious diseases. Take chicken pox, for example, a virus that eludes your innate immune system to create its characteristic blisters and itchy rash. But once you've been exposed, chicken pox is so effectively handled by your adaptive immune system that you'll probably get it only once, during childhood. At least that's how it was when I was young. Now that there is a vaccine available, many people don't get chicken pox at all. Vaccines are another example of your adaptive immune system at work; they use weakened, inactive, or simulated versions of viruses to teach your adaptive immune system how to fight the pathogen more effectively. Think of the COVID-19 vaccine, which teaches the adaptive immune system how to deal with a serious novel pathogen, so vaccinated people get COVID at lower rates, and those who do get it have a much lower chance of serious symptoms.[8]

The adaptive immune system is called into action by the innate immune system through antigen-presenting cells. These cells—particularly dendritic cells, named for their branching structure—detect and identify antigens, a general term for small, harmful molecules of foreign substances that can trigger an immune response. When an antigen is detected, antigen-presenting cells activate T cells, a type of white blood cell that is a major player in adaptive immunity. When activated, T cells differentiate into helper T cells and killer T cells. Helper T cells offer support by secreting cytokines that coordinate the immune response in a variety of ways. Killer T cells destroy cells that have been corrupted. T cells are assisted by B cells, another type of white blood cell that is tasked with producing antibodies. Antibodies are proteins that bind to antigens, neutralizing threats and eliminating them from your body.

The signature of the adaptive immune system is that both T cells and B cells get better at their jobs with time. Each exposure they have to a particular pathogen sharpens their response, leading to a more effective defense the next time they fight it. Your body remembers which antibodies to produce for different antigens, so challenges to your immune system are much more easily met. And if your immune system doesn't have to work as hard to protect you, it will be easier for you to feel your best. What might have been a debilitating illness the first time your body encounters it might be something you don't even notice the next time you fight it off.

I want to emphasize that this is a bare-bones overview of the mechanics of your immune system. The field of immunology is extremely complex, and research continues to uncover new aspects. But just knowing the basics is enough to understand the ways in which your brain and gut can disrupt this intricate machine.

IMMUNITY AND YOUR GUT

There are few things I love more than holding a newborn baby. It's so incredible to imagine how what started as a mere zygote nine months before has become a living, breathing infant, so full of the beautiful potential to grow and develop all the incredibly complex systems that make up our bodies. In addition to marveling over tiny hands and feet, I can't help but imagine the development of a fledgling gut microbiome.

While other major parts of the baby's body would have developed during the mother's pregnancy, the microbiome doesn't have the same head start. Babies in utero are largely sterile, with the mother's body keeping potentially harmful microbes far from a developing fetus (though there has been recent research indicating the presence of some bacteria in the placenta, umbilical cord, and amniotic fluid). Once the baby emerges into the world, however, there's no such luxury—even a young infant needs the benefits of a friendly gut microbiome and a robust immune system to protect against invaders. Though the microbiome isn't passed down genetically and doesn't develop in the womb, a mother still has ways to help her new baby establish a colony of helpful bacteria.[9]

The first vector for helping a baby develop a microbiome is in the birth canal. As the baby passes through during a vaginal birth, the mother confers bacteria from her intestines and vagina; these bacteria form the basis of the microbiome. Premature babies and those delivered by C-section miss out on that initial transfer, resulting in less complex microbiomes than those of babies delivered vaginally at full term. This is a necessary trade-off, since C-sections are often essential for the health of mother and baby, and the difference in microbiome composition gradually recedes, with most babies having similar bacterial composition at around a year old. Still, adults who were delivered by C-section have been shown to have an increased risk of infections, allergies, and inflammatory disorders.[10]

There is an explosion of good bacteria in the first week of the baby's life, facilitated by breastfeeding, which promotes a healthy microbiome and growing immunity through the transfer of antibodies.[11] As different strains of bacteria proliferate, they spur the development of different features of the immune system. For example, in the first hours after birth, a baby's microbiome largely consists of strains like Enterobacteriaceae that promote the development of natural killer cells and other types of T cells. In the first week of life, the vast increase in bacterial proliferation leads to the development of new types of leukocytes, like neutrophils and macrophages. In the following weeks, as strains like Firmicutes and Bacteroidetes take over, leukocytes mature and B cells develop. Finally, both systems gradually reach maturity at around two years old, but any disruption in that gut-immune development process can mean trouble later in life.[12] The use of microbiome-disrupting antibiotics in childhood can lead to issues with antibodies and cytokines that lead to increased susceptibility to allergies and asthma.[13] Certain differences in gut microbiome composition can lead to childhood disorders like type 1 diabetes[14] and to long-term metabolic disorders like obesity, type 2 diabetes, and nonalcoholic fatty liver disease (we'll learn more about metabolic disorders in chapter 6).[15]

I want to be clear that C-section delivery, formula feeding, and using antibiotics to fight serious infection during infancy are all important and valuable tools that help ensure that every baby can be born safely. Each mother's situation is different. Our growing knowledge about the role of the gut microbiome in immune development isn't a reason to discourage those practices, but rather a reason to develop new ways to mitigate the trade-offs as effectively as possible. Happily, ongoing research has shown real promise in the potential of probiotic treatments to help spur healthy microbiome and immune development in these cases.[16]

Even if your microbiome and immune system were healthy during their formation, that's no guarantee that everything will continue to function perfectly. Throughout your whole life, your gut microbiota and your immune system will continue to work together and keep each other in balance, nowhere more crucially than in the gut mucosa.

YOUR BODY'S MOST IMPORTANT LINE OF DEFENSE

While the immune system is active throughout the body, immune cells particularly like to hang out in the gut. In chapter 2, we learned that the gut contains the largest collection of nerve cells in the body; not to be outdone, 70–80 percent of your immune cells reside in your gut as well![17]

That concentration of immune cells makes sense when you consider the challenge your gut faces every day. The food you eat is full of vital nutrients, but it can also carry dangerous pathogens — the kinds of harmful bacteria, viruses, and parasites that might lead to various forms of food poisoning, like norovirus, salmonella, staph, listeria, and botulism. The digestive process brings those potentially harmful invaders deep into your body, where they must be contained to keep from causing you harm. Your gut separates out the helpful nutrients while rejecting harmful bacteria and other pathogens, ideally neutralizing the threats and ejecting them as waste. But your gut can't afford to be indiscriminate, rejecting all bacteria on sight. As we well know, to function properly the gut relies on massive colonies of helpful bacteria, which must be preserved even as harmful bacteria are destroyed. Separating the good bacteria from the bad bacteria is a tall order, and it's possible only thanks to a huge variety of processes and methods of communication between your immune system and your gut.[18]

The nexus of immune action in the gut is the intestinal mucosa, a layer of mucus lined by epithelial cells, which provides a barrier between the potentially harmful contents of your gut and the rest of your body.[19] If you look at a cross section of the small intestine, you'll see a cylindrical tube that looks like a roll of paper towels. The layers of paper towel are the outer layers of the gut, made up mostly of different types of muscle that help your body squeeze food through your intestinal tract. The hollow middle of the tube, the intestinal lumen, is where most of your gut microbiota reside. The cardboard that makes up the walls of the tube is the intestinal mucosa. The immune system sets up shop in the mucosa, keeping a close eye to make sure no threats arise. In fact, in a healthy gut, *all* immune response takes place in the mucosa, because harmful bacteria are not able to penetrate through this protective layer into the rest of your body.[20]

When everything is functioning well and your gut health is properly balanced, with helpful bacteria protected and harmful bacteria contained, you have achieved gut homeostasis. But if you have an imbalance in your gut bacteria leading to an overgrowth of bad bacteria, or if something goes awry in your immune system, this crucial interaction in your gut mucosa can break down. The mucosa itself can physically degrade and become easier to penetrate, allowing harmful pathogens to slip through into the rest of your body. This is the dreaded leaky gut (more formally called intestinal permeability) that is increasingly recognized as an enemy of good mental and physical health.[21] While we are only at the beginning of our understanding of the array of harm that can be caused by leaky gut, increased intestinal permeability has been linked with an increase in many different conditions, from gastric ulcers to food allergies to metabolic diseases like diabetes, autoimmune diseases like inflammatory bowel disease (IBD) and celiac, chronic inflammation, and cancer.[22] As we'll see in chapter 4, leaky gut is a key cause of increased inflammation throughout the body, another major factor in anxiety.

I want to emphasize that none of these interactions are taking place in a vacuum. As we discussed in chapter 2, gut dysbiosis can be fuel for anxiety on its own. And now we understand that gut dysbiosis can also drive immune disruption, which can trigger or worsen anxiety in other ways. In other words, any factor that upsets gut health or immune health is likely to upset mental health, too. It's all connected.

For now, let's turn our focus away from the gut to the rest of the body to see some direct links between mental health and immunity that illustrate how being anxious can make you sick, and how being sick can make you anxious.

THE CONNECTION BETWEEN IMMUNITY AND ANXIETY

My patient Eileen seemed happy. Everyone at work called her "Miss Sunshine." Others would complain when things got busy and stressful, but Eileen kept on smiling. She smiled through everything at work and at home: her toxic boss, her unsupportive husband, and her overwhelming life. Even when she came to my office for help with her "work stress," she was reluctant to drop the facade. It took several months to get her to open up about her overwhelm, but eventually she started to talk to me about how difficult things had truly been for her. When a big project came up at work, she was tasked with holding everything together, managing personalities and heavy workloads under tight deadlines. Those stressful periods were particularly challenging for her, but even between projects when work was quiet, she talked about how she was constantly full of dread, a feeling she tried to bury down deep. My suspicions were confirmed: Eileen was suffering from anxiety.

I began to help Eileen identify and understand the layers of her anxiety through therapy, trying to help her manage the busy periods and let go of her dread between projects. But even as she worked on her mental health, something else began to concern me. She started to lose weight, despite not trying to do so. Anxiety can cause some people to lose their appetite, but that hadn't been the case for Eileen in the past. I encouraged her to get evaluated by her primary care doctor, who in turn referred her to a specialist. Before long, she was diagnosed with breast cancer.

As a cancer thriver myself, I understood the crushing weight of the diagnosis, but I also knew that Eileen had the resilience and strength necessary to regain her health. It made me reflect on how my experience with cancer helped me become more in tune with my spiritual practice and mindfulness and led me to the principles of nutritional psychiatry, which became the blueprint of my work today. Little did I know at that point that those practices of sound nutrition were also positively impacting my immunity.

Thankfully, as scary as it was, Eileen's cancer was manageable, and she responded well to chemotherapy. After her recovery, she continued to embody a positive and upbeat attitude, but together we developed strategies to help her avoid suppressing her emotions to such a dramatic and destructive degree, and we made changes in her diet to help quell anxiety and support her immunity.

There's no way to determine the direct cause of Eileen's cancer. There are a host of factors involved in breast cancer, and any number of them could have been at play. But I have a hunch that Eileen's mental health played a role in leaving her more susceptible to cancer. A 2019 review of fifty-one studies, encompassing a sample of 2,611,907 participants over a mean time period of more than ten years, established that people diagnosed with depression and/or anxiety were significantly more likely to get cancer, with higher rates of mortality from cancer as well.[23]

Regardless of whether Eileen's personality traits contributed to her cancer, there is abundant evidence that our emotions can affect our immunity. For instance, an interesting cross-sectional study from 2022 showed that patients who suffered from mental illnesses like anxiety and depression had a higher risk of severe complications from COVID-19 than patients who had no such history.[24]

It doesn't take a team of medical researchers to guess that you're more likely to get sick when you are suffering from stress and anxiety, nor is it difficult to see why suffering from an illness might cause a strain on your mental health. We've all had those moments when our immune systems seem to break down at the worst moments, just as life is disrupted by major happenings at work or at home. But unlike a lot of folklore about susceptibility to illness—for instance, that being caught in the rain will lead to a cold, which my beloved grandma would tell me all the time—this one is actually true! And luckily for us, there *are* teams of medical researchers in the field of psychoneuroimmunology dedicated to understanding this very connection.

HOW DOES MENTAL HEALTH AFFECT THE IMMUNE SYSTEM?

Eileen's struggles with her mental health were rooted in two separate but related issues: stress and anxiety. As we discussed in chapter 1, the two conditions are tightly related, and they trigger the same response in your brain and body, but there are key distinctions between them. Stress is caused by an external trigger; in Eileen's case it was the big work projects that she handled well on the surface but that took a toll on her mind and body. Stress can cause an array of symptoms in your brain and body, including irritability, upset stomach, and disrupted sleep. But ideally, when the source of the stress is removed, the symptoms disappear. Anxiety results in symptoms similar to those caused by stress, but as we discussed in chapter 1, it is rooted internally, persisting even when there is nothing concrete to be anxious about. Eileen's stress was certainly feeding her anxiety, but even during easier periods at work she couldn't feel calm; she was stuck in a state of constant dread that kept her body's stress response firing no matter what was actually going on at work.

Remember that stress exerts its impact on the immune system via the CNS; the ANS, which controls our fight-or-flight response; and the HPA-axis. The HPA-axis regulates the release of crucial hormones, particularly the "stress hormone" cortisol, which spikes when your body is under acute stress to give you an extra jolt of energy. While cortisol and other similar hormones like epinephrine (also known as adrenaline) play an important role in keeping you safe from danger, too much of them can have a variety of negative effects, including weight gain, fatigue, and high blood pressure. They can also dysregulate the immune system, interfering with the production of various cytokines that help you respond to threats.[25]

I want to reiterate that hormones released in the stress response aren't necessarily bad — without our ability to react strongly in stressful situations, I'm sure our species would have been considerably less successful! And there's even some evidence that acute stress can actually stimulate the immune system. For example, studies have shown that short-term stress can enhance immune responses induced by vaccines and triggered by fighting tumors and recovering from surgery.[26] Other studies have shown that acute stress enhances the function of immune cells in both innate and adaptive immune responses.[27]

But in other cases, even acute stress can be harmful to your immune system. For example, a decade-long study of medical students found that the students' immunity went down every year under the simple stress of the three-day exam period. Test takers had fewer natural killer cells, they almost stopped producing the immunity-boosting cytokine gamma interferon, and their infection-fighting T cells showed a weaker than normal response. For stress of any significant duration — from a few days to a few months or years — all aspects of immunity went downhill.[28]

Treating Eileen helped me understand why it is so critical for anxiety sufferers to know a little more about these connections. While acute stress can have positive and negative effects, researchers agree that long-term stress is universally harmful to the immune system. A review of more than three hundred studies spanning thirty years found that chronic stress causes significant damage to nearly all measures of the immune system, including leukocyte counts, natural killer cell function, and cytokine production.[29] This is because cortisol and other chemicals released by the stress response are not intended to linger in your system. They're designed to give you a quick burst of energy to get you out of harm's way, after which the threat should be averted and the stress response can dissipate. But if the stress response is not turned off—either because of continuous exposure to actual stressors or because anxiety is tricking your brain into anticipating stressors that have not appeared yet—your immune system begins to lose the ability to fight inflammation and coordinate and communicate to respond to threats.[30] As a result, chronic stress has been linked with an elevated risk for numerous diseases, including infectious illnesses, cardiovascular disease, diabetes, certain cancers, and autoimmune disease, as well as general frailty and mortality.

Think back to Eileen. Before she came to see me, her cycle of stress and anxiety was never-ending. Even when she wasn't in an especially stressful period at work, her anxiety ensured that her brain kept the flood of cortisol and other stress hormones flowing, giving her immune system no chance to recover. Therefore, it's not surprising that anxiety disorders have also been specifically linked with this conflict between stress hormones, increased inflammation, and decreased immunity. For instance, one study found that people with GAD had imbalanced levels of crucial cytokines compared to the control group.[31] Another study showed that patients with GAD were more likely to develop cardiac disease or have heart attacks.[32] Other studies have suggested that GAD patients have reduced T cell activation compared to control groups.[33]

One of the clearest indications of the link between mental health and immunity is the incidence of autoimmune diseases in anxiety patients, just like we saw with Mary and her struggle with lupus at the beginning of the chapter. Autoimmune diseases are conditions where the body's immune system attacks healthy cells as if they were pathogens. Like lupus, most autoimmune diseases are chronic with no definitive cure, though symptoms can often be managed through a treatment plan. In a variety of studies, autoimmune conditions like lupus, multiple sclerosis, and rheumatoid arthritis have been shown to correlate with serious mental health conditions, from schizophrenia to psychosis,[34] and also more common conditions like stress and anxiety.[35]

While there is still much to learn about the connections between anxiety and immune disruption, we know enough to definitively say that this is yet another crucial link between mental health and whole-body health.

WRAPPING UP IMMUNITY AND ANXIETY

Now that you know more about the relationship between anxiety, your gut, and your immunity, I hope you can see the complexity of these problems and the difficulty of trying to pinpoint where things are going awry. But I want to emphasize again that it's not necessary to know where the issues begin, because no matter what, the most powerful treatment in all these areas is the food you eat. A proper, healthy diet will always result in a healthy microbiome, which will always boost immunity and calm your mind.

As we've touched on throughout this chapter, one of the most destructive effects of disrupted immunity is increased inflammation. In the next chapter, we'll focus on the dangers of chronic inflammation and how it is connected to anxiety.

CHAPTER FOUR

Inflammation on the Brain

A forty-nine-year-old man named Adi came to see me about a sudden case of anxiety that was taking over his life. Though Adi had never struggled with mental health before, he had recently begun experiencing panic attacks. He told me that when he walked his dog, every time they passed another dog in the neighborhood, his heart would race and his palms would become sweaty, his fingers feeling as though the leash was about to slip from his grasp. His mind raced with thoughts and images of his dog being attacked or running into traffic. He knew the fear wasn't rational. The other dogs were friendly, and his own was a well-trained, obedient, and loving companion. His anxiety was creeping into his work life as well. Sunday nights and Monday mornings were particularly bad, as he pictured a multitude of crises that loomed, disasters that would surely lead to him being fired. Again, he knew these feelings weren't warranted, because he had worked at his job for decades and was a valued member of the team.

His panic attacks had become so bad that much of his day was spent worrying about whether he was going to have another one. As much as they had colored his existence, he emphasized that he did not want to be on medication, but he was determined to find other strategies to stop these troubling mental episodes before they became a way of life.

What Is a Panic Attack?

A panic attack is an event when you might experience four or more of the following symptoms: sweating, trembling, unsteadiness, derealization (feeling as if you're in a dream or trance), elevated heart rate, nausea, tingling, shortness of breath, fear of dying, fear of going crazy, chills, choking, or chest pain.

Even if you recover quickly from a panic attack, you should seek professional help. Panic attacks can recur unexpectedly, and panic disorder often overlaps with unemployment, depression, substance abuse, and suicidal thoughts.[1] Additionally, if you feel symptoms like chest pain, you will need professional assessment in an emergency room or urgent care to determine whether you are having a heart attack. Even if you think it's a panic attack, it's better to err on the side of caution.

When I talked to him about his change in mood, he conjectured that it might be that he was approaching his fiftieth birthday, which had sparked some fears about aging and mortality. He also told me that his mother had passed away a year before, which left a gaping hole in his life. He had never married, and the two of them had lived alone together ever since his father passed away when he was just a teenager. He missed her love and companionship and was having trouble coming to terms with his grief.

As someone who has deep ties with my own family, I very much understood the pain that Adi was going through, and I would never discount the mental burden that such a great loss can have on a person. Even though he said the rawest feelings of grief had passed, and he was insistent that his panic attacks didn't feel directly connected to his emotions about his mother's death, we discussed how the pain of loss was creating a major obstacle in his ability to fully move on with his life.

I also suspected something else was at play. After speaking with Adi further, I learned that his mother's death not only had caused a change in his security and support system but had also meant a major shift in his diet. Adi told me that he had always helped with chores around the house and food shopping but that his mother had done all the cooking. Since her death, his old routines felt painful, so he had largely stopped shopping for food, and even when he did, he found himself at a loss for how to turn the healthy ingredients into the wholesome meals his mother had made. Adrift, Adi had lapsed into a cycle of relying on takeout and sweets to soothe himself.

Taking stock of his diet, and coordinating it with the onset of his anxiety, I was worried that Adi's problem was being worsened by chronic inflammation. I talked to him about the dangers of a pro-inflammatory diet and how his body was likely sending constant signals to muster an immune response to a threat that wasn't going away, leaving his brain in disarray. Adi's insurance didn't cover blood tests for inflammation, but I assured him we didn't need to perform them. We simply needed to get his diet back under control, emphasizing anti-inflammatory foods that would break the cycle of an out-of-control immune response and let his body and brain regain stability.

Since we had such a clear timeline of his shift in diet and the onset of his symptoms, Adi's treatment plan was simple. He limited his intake of refined sugars and the processed vegetable oils often used by fast-food chains. To encourage himself to switch back to home-cooked meals, he enrolled in cooking classes, giving him an opportunity to socialize and make friends while learning how to cook new dishes, along with some of the old favorites his mom had made. Quickly, Adi began to see cooking as a form of therapy, nourishing but also relaxing. It became a way to stimulate new learning, honor his mother's legacy, and absorb the love and care she had imparted through cooking.

After three months, Adi started to notice that he felt profoundly better. He'd had no panic attacks, and his worry had decreased substantially. He learned how to cook three meals that he could rotate, and how to build a healthy salad when time was short. He developed strategies for meal prep so that he would never be tempted to grab fast food on his lunch break at work. He joined an online cooking club and continued to go to cooking classes, forming a community that helped fend off the loneliness. He bought a tread-mill and began exercising regularly. Slowly but surely, he made peace with the loss of his mother and was able to feel like his old self, getting back to a more relaxed state of mind.

By understanding chronic inflammation, we can see how inter-woven the relationships between diet, immune system, and anxiety are. In a 2010 review, psychoneuroimmunologist Janice Kiecolt-Glaser outlined just how tightly knit these processes can be, with anxiety fueling poor diet choices, poor diet choices leading to greater inflam-mation, and inflammation driving further anxiety.[2] In this chapter, we'll untangle these complicated relationships and learn another way to calm your mind with food.

WHAT IS INFLAMMATION?

I'm sure you've heard about the ill effects of inflammation. In recent years, inflammation has ascended the hierarchy of medical threats to achieve buzzword status. On morning shows, in books, and of course across the internet and social media, you will find a deluge of advice about how to fight inflammation in your body. There's good reason for that heightened attention, because chronic inflam-matory diseases like heart disease, stroke, and diabetes together are the most common cause of death worldwide. The World Health Organization estimates that 74 percent of all deaths and 86 percent of deaths before age seventy are owing to noncommunicable dis-eases, many of which are deeply connected to inflammation.[3] And recent research is showing us that inflammation is a key factor in mental health conditions, too.

Thanks to the amount of discussion surrounding inflammation, when I talk about it with my patients, I can trust that they have at least some familiarity with the concept. But I often find that they get a bit overwhelmed trying to balance everything they've heard. Inflammation is such a big topic and can cause so many different types of harm to the body that it can be confusing to parse the specifics. I feel strongly that people need to understand the real health impact underlying the buzzwords so they can meaningfully integrate the information to improve their mental well-being.

It's easy enough to understand that inflammation is *bad,* but it takes a bit more effort to understand all the reasons why. Part of the reason for the confusion is that inflammation *isn't* always bad. In fact, the kind of inflammation that you're likely most familiar with is actually good—even if it doesn't feel that way. The redness, swelling, and pain you suffer following an injury—whether a paper cut, a bug bite, or a twisted ankle—are all signs of so-called acute inflammation. As we touched on in chapter 3, acute inflammation is one of the immune system's most commonly used tools to help it do its job. Inflammation causes blood vessels to dilate, allowing more blood flow to the injured tissue, bringing with it a flood of white blood cells and making conditions hostile to invading pathogens. It also confers a variety of advantages to immune cells and promotes healing in other ways. In addition to healing injuries, acute inflammation is also useful in the fight against disease. Any disease that ends in the suffix "-itis" causes inflammation in some way. That might mean an inflamed eye, as in conjunctivitis (the dreaded "pink eye"); inflamed airways, as in bronchitis; or inflamed skin, as in dermatitis.

Acute inflammation almost always causes pain, itchiness, or other discomfort. Consequently, treating an illness or injury that is causing acute inflammation often means trying to reduce that inflammation to make you feel better—for example, putting ice on a twisted ankle to bring down the swelling—but inflammation is still a crucial part of the body's reparative process. Most importantly, it's temporary. Once your immune system heals the problem, either on its own or through medical treatment, the inflammation abates and your body can return to normal function.

But what if inflammation doesn't go away? Your twisted ankle or paper cut will heal easily enough, but other conditions are more difficult for your body to solve, prolonging the duration of the inflammatory response. When it lingers for months or years, it's considered chronic and becomes much more insidious and destructive. Chronic inflammation is a silent killer. Though some chronic inflammatory conditions come with obvious symptoms—for example, the painful swollen joints of rheumatoid arthritis or the gastrointestinal difficulties of Crohn's disease—most do not. You often don't know that you're suffering from chronic inflammation until you have a heart attack or stroke or develop a serious inflammatory condition that can be difficult to treat. As we saw in Adi's case, the onset of chronic inflammation can also bring on symptoms of anxiety, like the panic attacks he started suffering after a lifetime of reliable mental health.

Chronic inflammation has a variety of causes. Sometimes it results from a bacterial or fungal infection that didn't quite get eradicated and lingers in tissues, continually sparking an immune response, like we see in chronic fatigue syndrome. Sometimes it's caused by autoimmune conditions like lupus, which we discussed in chapter 3, as the body misfires and attacks its own tissues. It can be caused by continued exposure to environmental toxins or substances the body is allergic to.[4] And, as we saw with Adi, it can be caused by continued exposure to unhealthy foods through poor dietary choices, an association we'll dig into later in the chapter.

Regardless of its cause, chronic inflammation can wreak significant damage on your body. Constantly marshaling an ineffective immune response takes a lot of energy to sustain, which pulls resources away from your body's core tasks and spreads your immune system thin. Furthermore, your organs are not meant to withstand the harshness of inflammatory responses for extended periods of time. What is designed to be a tool to help your body heal becomes a destructive force, and your own white blood cells damage your tissues. Over time, this damage can accumulate into a root cause of metabolic syndrome (which we will discuss in greater detail in chapter 6), heart disease, cancer, neurodegenerative diseases like Alzheimer's, and as we will learn in this chapter, mental health conditions like anxiety.[5]

TESTING FOR INFLAMMATION

Since we can't necessarily see or feel chronic inflammation, the surest way to confirm its existence is through a blood test that measures levels of inflammatory markers, compounds that show up in the blood during inflammatory responses. Many prominent markers are different types of cytokines, the immune system's messengers we learned about in chapter 3. One of the most commonly cited is interleukin-6, a type of cytokine that sends warnings about pathogens throughout the body.[6] Non-cytokine inflammatory markers include proteins such as C-reactive protein, which is produced in the liver and is a valuable inflammatory marker in many studies involving anxiety.[7]

Blood tests for inflammation are not regularly performed as part of traditional blood panels, though they are increasingly common among integrative and functional medicine practitioners, and they are used widely for inflammation research. There is disagreement about their usefulness in the medical community — though they can confirm the presence of inflammation, they don't help specify what's *causing* the inflammation, nor do they differentiate between acute and chronic inflammation. In other words, even if a test for inflammatory markers comes back positive, there is still guesswork involved to determine the cause and scope of the inflammation.

My approach is always to bridge the gap between clinical presentation and lab data as sensibly as possible. There are many situations in which "test, don't guess" is the correct approach — for example, if I suspect a patient might have a vitamin deficiency, I would always order a test. However, as we saw with Adi, inflammation tests are rarely necessary, especially since the type of dietary interventions I recommend are a low-risk treatment. Rather than repeating costly blood tests that may not give a definitive answer, I always find it's better for a patient to make dietary changes and see how symptoms respond.

INFLAMMATION AND ANXIETY

Take a moment to reflect on what we've learned about inflammation: a protective process persists even in the absence of threats, wreaking havoc on the body it's supposed to safeguard. Does that dilemma feel familiar? It should, because it's the same basic pattern we learned about anxiety in chapter 1. Chronic inflammation is sustained immune response in the absence of an acute cause. Anxiety is sustained fear response in the absence of a tangible threat. In other words, both are functions of the body's own defenses going overboard and causing harm.

Of course, more significant than that philosophical link is the hard scientific evidence that the two are tightly connected. The simplest indication of a link is that numerous studies have shown that patients suffering from a variety of anxiety disorders have high levels of inflammatory markers. For instance, a 2018 review of forty-one studies found that anxiety sufferers had higher levels of pro-inflammatory cytokines than healthy controls.[8] A 2019 review found that GAD patients had significantly higher levels of C-reactive protein than healthy controls.[9] A 2022 study showed the same association in GAD patients as well as in people with panic disorders.[10] And a 2021 study of 144,890 patients from a British database called the UK Biobank found similar results, with interleukin-6 and C-reactive protein levels elevated in patients with depression and anxiety.[11] Studies of depression have shown similar results.[12]

Correlation between anxiety and elevated inflammatory markers establishes a connection between the two conditions that is too consistent to be coincidence, but it doesn't say much about causality. Does anxiety cause inflammation? Or does inflammation cause anxiety? I doubt it will surprise you that our best evidence indicates that it's a two-way street.

There is evidence that inflammation in the body can ignite anxiety in the brain. In animal studies, researchers have performed tests where they have introduced inflammatory cytokines into mice. This influx of simulated inflammation causes the mice to display depressed and anxious behavior, which goes away when they are treated with anti-inflammatory cytokines.[13] Human studies have shown that inflammation related to sickness can drive shifts in mood, including depression and anxiety, among other negative consequences that researchers call "sickness behavior."[14]

On the other hand, as we established in chapter 3, chronic stress response is recognized as one of the primary causes of inflammation.[15] We've already learned how stress chemicals such as cortisol and adrenaline can be helpful in the short term but harmful when present for long periods at high levels. Sure enough, chronic, persistent stress response has been identified as a cause of chronic inflammation.[16] And as we know, while stress and anxiety aren't identical, anxiety can worsen and prolong the bad effects of stressful periods. Furthermore, negative emotions like anxiety have been shown to contribute to a slower wound-healing process, leading to a greater risk of prolonged inflammation.[17] And mental health issues have also been associated with increased production of inflammatory cytokines in the absence of other sources of inflammation.[18] In other words, an anxious brain can cause or worsen inflammation in the body.

Though there is clearly robust research confirming these relationships between inflammation and mental health, we're still in the very early stages of fully understanding the exact pathways through which inflammation worsens anxiety (and vice versa). Through imaging studies that monitor the way the brain reacts in the presence of inflammatory cytokines, researchers have found that inflammatory markers can lead to neurotransmitter imbalances, decreasing important chemicals like serotonin, dopamine, and GABA. That's similar to how gut dysbiosis can lead to shortfalls in those same chemicals, knocking brain chemistry out of proper balance. Furthermore, inflammation in the CNS can increase the responsiveness of the amygdala—which, as we established in chapter 1, is a central nexus of anxiety—along with the responsiveness of other parts of the brain that play a role in mood and threat response.[19]

Given these connections, there is certainly great potential for future therapies that reduce inflammation as a method of treating anxiety and other mental health conditions.[20] In fact, some researchers believe that the anti-inflammatory effects of SSRIs such as fluoxetine (Prozac) and escitalopram (Lexapro) may play a role in how they work on anxiety.[21] Even anti-inflammatory drugs that aren't designed to treat mental health problems can have a positive effect. Consider a 2020 study on the effectiveness of the familiar anti-inflammatory aspirin on mental health issues in cancer patients. Among a cohort of 316,904 patients with a cancer diagnosis, 5,613 patients received a diagnosis of depression, anxiety, or stress-related disorder one year after their cancer diagnosis. However, the researchers found that patients who had already been regularly taking aspirin (usually as a preventative for a heart attack or stroke) had a significantly lower rate of anxiety and depression than those who had not.[22]

I don't mean to suggest that everyone suffering from anxiety should immediately start taking aspirin, because even seemingly harmless over-the-counter drugs can come with complications and side effects (for example, daily aspirin use thins your blood and can lead to gastrointestinal bleeding). It will take further research to pinpoint the exact nature of the connections between anxiety and inflammation to determine the efficacy and safety of treatments built around anti-inflammatory pharmaceuticals.

What we already know, however, is that one of the primary drivers of chronic inflammation is eating a poor diet. And one of the best ways to reduce inflammation is to eat a healthy diet full of anti-inflammatory foods. Thus, if eating poorly aggravates inflammation, and inflammation worsens anxiety, eating an anti-inflammatory diet will fight anxiety. Before we dive into the ways in which food can worsen inflammation, I want to highlight one more specific type of inflammation that is a particular threat to mental health.

THE DANGERS OF NEUROINFLAMMATION

Thus far, we've been discussing chronic inflammation that can arise anywhere in your body — so-called peripheral inflammation in medical literature. But there is a specific type of inflammation that has special relevance to your brain: neuroinflammation. Just like it sounds, neuroinflammation is inflammation centered in your CNS, which consists of your brain and spinal cord. Unlike your digestive tract, which is well equipped to deal with invading microbes that tag along in your food, your CNS is not designed to have contact with dangerous pathogens. That means that neuroinflammation is a very serious reaction, a last-ditch effort to protect your brain from harm.

Like inflammation elsewhere in your body, inflammation in the CNS starts out as a coordinated response to ward off harmful intruders. The most important immune soldiers in your nervous system are oval-shaped cells called microglia, which perform several roles in neuroimmunity, including surveillance for threats, production of cytokines, and the macrophage-like work of gobbling up harmful pathogens and damaged cells. When they sense something is awry, microglia can marshal a powerful inflammatory response to help correct the problem.[23]

Like inflammation in other parts of the body, this inflammatory response can be harmful as well as helpful, especially when it persists over long periods. Just as we saw with acute inflammation, in an ideal world, once the threat is neutralized, the inflammatory response is turned off and the neurons of your CNS can go back to their everyday tasks of helping you think, feel, know, move, respond, and react. If neuroinflammation grows unchecked because of chronic exposure to toxins or crossed wires in your immune system, serious problems can arise.

As we saw with peripheral inflammation, stress has been shown to be a major source of neuroinflammation, aggravating microglia in the amygdala, hippocampus, and other anxiety centers.[24] Microglial activation has been associated with anxiety,[25] depression,[26] and a host of serious neurological disorders, including Alzheimer's disease, Parkinson's disease, multiple sclerosis, and amyotrophic lateral sclerosis.[27] Again, this is a very new field of research, and I have a feeling we are only scratching the surface of understanding the full threat of neuroinflammation.

Interestingly, recent research has shown that diet can have a real impact on levels of neuroinflammation, potentially decreasing anxiety as well as the risk of other long-term neurological conditions. Rather than focusing on the foods you eat, this research has focused on *when* you eat that food, studying the effects of dietary restriction, through either reducing the amount of food you eat per day or limiting the time frames in which you eat.[28] We'll talk more about the possibilities for implementing an intermittent fasting plan in chapter 11.

HOW FOOD PROMOTES INFLAMMATION

When I was in medical school, I had a friend who was allergic to peanuts. At the time, I remember being surprised at her level of constant vigilance to make sure she never came in contact with them. She avoided almost all baked goods, knowing that even if a cookie didn't directly contain peanuts, there was the possibility of cross-contamination in the kitchen. She wouldn't live with roommates unless they agreed not to have peanuts or peanut butter in the house. She carried her EpiPen in her lab coat pocket even when we were on clinical duties with no peanuts or other snacks in sight.

Though I respected her diligence at protecting herself so thoroughly, I didn't fully understand the difficulty of her position until I devoted my career to understanding the devastating effects of making the wrong dietary choices. It can be deeply frightening to understand that something as simple and pleasurable as eating could have deadly side effects. And while most of us don't have severe food allergies, understanding them can help shed light on why our bodies reject other harmful types of food as well.

Food is made up of the same fundamental building blocks as we are. Your digestive process reduces food down to these basics in order to convert them to nutrients and energy. However, some people's bodies mistakenly recognize some of these compounds as toxic and attempt to reject them. The immune system alerts a special cell called a mast cell, which stores and then releases an immune chemical called histamine. Histamine can cause a variety of allergic symptoms, most of which involve increasing inflammation. And as we've learned in this chapter, increased inflammation means increased anxiety.

In that sense, food allergies can cause anxiety in two ways: Food-allergic people can develop anxieties surrounding their efforts to avoid the foods that pose a threat. And having an allergic reaction to food can be a driver of chronic inflammation, which also drives anxiety. Furthermore, food allergy–related inflammation has been directly implicated as a risk factor for neuroinflammation, resulting in an increase in microglia and the presence of inflammation markers in the brain.[29] So while we may associate severe food allergies with anaphylaxis and other serious (potentially deadly) symptoms, even less extreme food allergies may have a long-term effect on mental health.

Food allergies are fairly common in the United States, with more than 10 percent of US adults testing as food allergic, and almost 20 percent of adults self-reporting that they have a food allergy (some of this discrepancy may be the result of nonallergic food intolerance, or differences in the way both of these conditions are defined and measured).[30] Furthermore, over the last decade or so, rates of food allergies have increased significantly. While there is much scientific discussion about the reasons why allergies are becoming more prevalent, one factor appears to be the gut microbiome. As we established in chapter 3, the gut microbiome plays a crucial role in the development of the immune system, and researchers have established that people with food allergies have different microbiome makeups than those without.[31]

The gut microbiome is also central to inflammation in those without food allergies. Given the interplay of gut microbiota, the immune system, and mental health, it's unsurprising that the gut has been found to mediate inflammatory responses. As we've seen in other contexts, the makeup of bacteria in the microbiome has a profound influence on whether the gut is a pro-inflammatory or anti-inflammatory environment. A 2021 study established that a gut-healthy diet of mostly plant-based food and fish led to lower levels of inflammation than a gut-unhealthy diet of processed food, unhealthy forms of animal-derived fats, and sugar. The healthier diet led to flourishing species of bacteria that assist in the production of SCFAs and increased levels of nutrient metabolism. The unhealthy diet led to overgrowth of bacteria that create toxins that trigger immune response and increase inflammation.[32]

An overgrowth of bad bacteria can also cause leaky gut syndrome, which we discussed in chapter 3. Remember that leaky gut occurs when the mucosal lining of your gut is damaged by toxins and becomes permeable because of an imbalance in your gut microbiome, allowing harmful pathogens to slip through. Once they are loose within your body, the immune system has to scramble to try to contain them before they can cause harm—once again, increasing inflammation is often a first line of defense. But if your gut microbiome is constantly out of balance, leading to a leaky gut that can't patch itself up, your body is going to be facing a steady stream of harmful pathogens. In other words, the stage is set for chronic inflammation and anxiety.

ANTI-INFLAMMATORY IS ANTIANXIETY

Just as the past decade has yielded an explosion of understanding about the links between gut health and mental health, I suspect the next ten years will continue to unpack the association between inflammation and anxiety. As our understanding of both conditions continues to grow, I am sure researchers will continue to break ground on how we can fight anxiety through treating inflammation— not to mention the vast array of inflammatory syndromes that threaten our health. But for now, the very best thing you can do to limit inflammation is to structure your diet in a way that avoids pro-inflammatory foods and prioritizes anti-inflammatory foods.

We will get into the specifics of eating an anti-inflammatory diet in part 2, but for the next two chapters, I want to turn our focus to the beginning and end of the digestive process to see further links between diet and anxiety. First we'll discuss leptin, a hormone that is key to regulating food intake and appetite. Then we'll explore your metabolism and learn how your body creates energy out of the food you eat—and how those processes can go wrong in a way that is a profound threat to mental health.

CHAPTER FIVE

Anxiety and Leptin, the Appetite Hormone

We've all had those stressful days at work. From the moment you first check your email, probably before you even get out of bed, everything you had planned for your entire day slips away from you. You spend hours at work putting out fires and dealing with irascible people. You know your performance is slipping with each unfortunate task, but there's no choice except to push through.

At the end of the day, you feel ineffective, exhausted, and at your wits' end. You realize you never ate or left your work-from-home space except to use the bathroom. You flop on the couch, stare at the ceiling, and hear your heart racing as you wait for your brain and body to calm down. As you lie there, you start to think of dinner and a bottle of wine—a glass just isn't going to cut it. In the kitchen, you open your pantry and try to decide what to eat. You see a box of instant mac and cheese, but you've been trying to lose weight and you know you shouldn't eat a huge bowl of refined carbs and fats.

Just when you've made up your mind to eat a healthy salad, a text pings on your phone. It's your boss, asking if you can jump on a call an hour later. No explanation, no assurances that everything is okay. Your mind shifts into overdrive. What is this about? It must be something important. What news could be bad enough that it can't wait until the next day? Are you being fired? Is corporate folding your department and laying everyone off? Even if there's no reason for panic, you're sick of how virtual work means there's no cutoff when you leave the office at five p.m.; work extends into all hours with no boundaries.

You look at the clock. An hour isn't much time, but suddenly it feels like an eternity, leaving your mind to stew about what your boss could want. At least you have some time to eat. You turn back to the pantry, but now eating responsibly doesn't feel like a priority. Out comes the mac and cheese, a baguette you can soak in garlic butter, and for good measure, a frozen pizza that you bought just because it was on sale. Before you know it, you've wolfed it all down, just in time to hear the ping of a text on your phone, causing your anxiety to spiral again. Your boss is ready for that call.

What went wrong? You were completely aware that you were making bad food choices, but suddenly, it was as if your brain had lost its ability to listen to reason, and something more instinctual took over. Part of the answer might be purely practical: you might rationalize to yourself that you only ate the junk food because it was easier or more convenient than healthier options. But there is another basic truth: stress and anxiety make you crave food, especially high-calorie, carb-, fat-, and sugar-laden comfort foods, which feel satiating in these moments. After all, they're called *comfort* foods for a reason, and scientific studies have confirmed that eating sugary, fatty food can lead to short-term improvement in mood during difficult emotional times.[1]

Medical researchers have studied that association through the study of a hormone called leptin. Since its discovery in 1994, leptin has become a centerpiece of research into our appetite, a vital link in understanding how our bodies and brains tell us when we are hungry and what to eat. The most recent research also points to leptin as another factor in the strong connections between anxiety and the food we eat.

WHAT IS LEPTIN?

Leptin is a hormone secreted by white adipose tissue, the medical term for the type of tissue that makes up most of an adult human's fat reserves. Though adipose tissue gets demonized in popular culture, a healthy human body requires a significant percentage of body fat to function properly. We used to think of adipose tissue as being largely inert, its purpose to insulate against cold temperatures and store excess calories, but recent research indicates that it's actually a full-fledged endocrine organ that secretes hormones that affect the entire body.[2] Leptin is one such hormone, and its main function is to signal to the brain when you've had enough to eat by inducing feelings of fullness, or satiety.

At its most basic, leptin acts as a kind of thermostat for your body's long-term energy-storage needs. Elevated levels of leptin reduce your appetite, and low levels of leptin increase your appetite. Therefore, if you have more adipose tissue — and therefore greater energy stores — more leptin is produced, telling your brain that you don't need to eat to excess. If you have less adipose tissue, less leptin is produced, signaling to your brain that your body needs to prioritize finding sustenance or risk starvation.

In performing this long-term management of fat stores, leptin also influences the amount of food you eat in a sitting, and even the type of foods you crave, particularly during stressful times. A variety of studies have shown that leptin levels are decreased following acute stress, which means that when you're stressed or anxious, your brain struggles to get the signal that you've had enough to eat.[3] Furthermore, studies have shown that lower leptin levels correlate with an urge to eat comfort food and that increased leptin during stressful times correlates with lower intake of comfort food.[4] And to complicate things even further, an overabundance of leptin as a result of being overweight can overwhelm leptin receptors, creating a condition called leptin resistance, which causes leptin to malfunction even when there is plenty to go around, making it even more difficult to change patterns of overeating.[5]

Given its key role in regulating appetite and food cravings, it's easy to see how disruptions in leptin can wreak havoc on the best-laid eating plans. And even beyond its core roles, science has uncovered more and more ways that leptin influences the body. We are now beginning to understand that leptin is a true head-to-toe hormone that has influence on the cardiovascular system, gastrointestinal system, renal system, immune system, and connective tissue.[6] But most significant is leptin's effect on your brain, which illustrates another key connection between food and anxiety.

Gender Differences in Leptin Concentration

After discovering leptin, one of the first things researchers learned is that women tend to have significantly higher serum leptin levels than men — usually three to four times higher. You might think this discrepancy is because of differences in adipose tissue, since women tend to have higher percentages of body fat than men. But the dichotomy persists across different weights and body fat percentages. Furthermore, women's brains appear to be more sensitive to the effects of leptin, and overweight men with abnormally high leptin levels are more likely than women to develop leptin resistance.[7]

There are theories about why this discrepancy exists — leptin levels in young and old men tend to be closer to those of women, so there is evidence that higher testosterone leads to lower leptin,[8] and differences in body composition mean that women are more likely to have more subcutaneous fat while men are more likely to have more visceral fat, which produces leptin at a lower rate[9] — but the important takeaway is that men may struggle more with leptin-related issues than women, whether because their leptin levels are naturally low, or because their brains become leptin-resistant.

The discrepancy also shapes leptin research, with many studies reporting different results for women and men, or focusing on only one gender at a time. Still, even if leptin affects the genders by different degrees, it plays the same basic role and has the same core effects on mental health in both men and women, so it's important for everyone to understand its influence.

LEPTIN AND ANXIETY

Building on everything we've learned so far in this book, it's not hard to predict the ways in which overeating, particularly binging on fats and sugars, can increase your anxiety—such a diet could very well lead to the kind of gut dysbiosis we learned about in chapter 2, which could upset the balance of brain chemistry, cause immune disruption as we saw in chapter 3, and lead to chronic inflammation as we saw in chapter 4. Once again, we see that all these systems are so tightly tied together that it can be difficult to pinpoint the exact cause of the problem.

But in addition to being a factor in poor diet choices, there is also growing evidence that leptin disruption could be directly involved in causing anxiety as well, because of how it affects the brain. Leptin's work to manage fat stores and regulate appetite involves a complicated signaling process that entails circulating from fat cells through the body as it monitors energy stores, and then transmitting that information to the brain to give instructions for regulating appetite. This information transfer in the brain happens via the brainstem, hypothalamus, and amygdala.[10] Remember from chapter 1 that the hypothalamus and amygdala are anxiety hot spots, controlling processes like reward and motivation, fear response, and fight-or-flight response.

Many studies have shown that proper leptin function has a calming effect on these parts of the brain, helping to alleviate anxiety. For example, animal studies have shown that increased leptin levels lead to a reduction in anxious behaviors on par with the results of the common antianxiety drug fluoxetine (Prozac).[11] Similar results have been found in humans, with studies in both men and women confirming that higher leptin levels correlate with lowered anxiety.[12]

Semaglutide is a medication sold under the brand names Ozempic and Wegovy. There is a lot of interest in and discussion about these medications for weight loss. Ozempic was approved in 2017 by the US Food and Drug Administration (FDA) for use in adults with type 2 diabetes.[13]

Ozempic is a weekly injection that helps lower blood sugar by helping the pancreas make more insulin. Wegovy is now approved for weight loss. You may wonder why I mention this in a chapter about leptin, but stay with me. When discussing leptin, it's important to mention Glucagon-like peptide (GLP-1) too. It is a hormone secreted by intestinal endocrine cells. GLP-1 inhibits food intake by inhibiting appetite.[14]

Ozempic acts like a GLP-1 receptor agonist — so it lowers fasting blood sugar, as well as blood sugar after we eat a meal, by stimulating insulin secretion. But Ozempic can also help improve leptin sensitivity and reduce leptin resistance. By activating the GLP-1 receptor, Ozempic can enhance the signaling of leptin in the brain, leading to a feeling of satiation and reduced hunger cravings.

A population-based study in Taiwan showed that those receiving GLP-1 receptor agonists for diabetes were at a significantly decreased risk for anxiety. This has anecdotally also been reported in the media. Although we are not at a point of prescribing these medications in mental health, it is helpful to know about this impact on anxiety. Last, by supporting your metabolic health and helping stabilize blood sugar levels, these medications may also indirectly help with anxiety.

On the other hand, lower leptin levels have been associated with a variety of anxiety disorders. For instance, in a study of patients suffering from panic disorder, subjects who had low leptin levels were more likely to suffer from panic attacks than those with higher leptin levels.[15] Low leptin levels have also been associated with GAD in men.[16] A similar association has been shown in patients suffering from obsessive-compulsive disorder and depression.[17] Animal studies have even suggested that leptin has the potential to reverse social anxiety, inducing greater trust and social interaction in mice.[18]

Since leptin is a compound produced inside your body, it's a challenge to "add more" via your diet. Still, if low leptin levels are causing issues with appetite and mental health, certain diet and lifestyle changes have been shown to increase leptin levels. For normal-weight individuals who are not leptin resistant, the best diets to follow are those high in healthy omega-3 fats, low in refined carbs and sugar, and full of fruits and vegetables. For instance, the Mediterranean diet, which we'll discuss in detail in chapter 11, is a great choice.

THE HIGHS AND LOWS OF LEPTIN

Thus far we've learned that leptin has an inverse relationship with anxiety: higher leptin means lower anxiety, and lower leptin means higher anxiety. While this association is true in most cases, it doesn't tell the whole story. In some cases, high serum leptin — that is, a large amount of leptin in your blood — can actually correlate with *higher* anxiety.

This positive association between leptin and anxiety is usually found in patients who are obese or otherwise struggling to control their appetite. For example, one study tracked leptin levels of breast cancer patients who were also suffering from anxiety. Out of two hundred participants, obese participants' leptin levels spiked more dramatically when they were anxious, which wasn't the case for nonobese subjects.[19] Another study showed that young people ages ten to sixteen who struggle to control their appetite also showed a positive relationship between anxiety and high serum leptin.[20] Several other studies have demonstrated that post-traumatic stress disorder is associated with a heightened risk of obesity and also higher serum levels of leptin.[21] And the fact that so many psychiatric drugs increase weight gain as a side effect exacerbates the leptin–anxiety problem.[22]

High levels of leptin are particularly associated with cases of "somatic anxiety," anxiety that manifests as physical symptoms without the accompanying mental symptoms. I once had a patient named Marguerite, a fifty-five-year-old single mother who had gone to her primary care physician because she'd been suffering from episodes of rapid breathing that appeared out of nowhere. She was overweight but otherwise healthy, and there was no obvious cause for her symptoms. After a battery of tests such as an electrocardiogram, lung X-rays, and blood work all came back clean, her primary care physician brought up the possibility that anxiety was causing her symptoms. Marguerite was understandably skeptical—she had never felt anxious before, and she hadn't noticed any obvious changes in her mental health alongside her breathing problems—but she agreed to see me to explore the possibility.

I explained to Marguerite that even if she didn't feel anxious, anxiety symptoms are expressed through the body ("somatic" means related to the body, distinct from the mind). They manifest as physical symptoms like the hyperventilation she was experiencing, as well as heart palpitations, frequent urination, dry mouth, and excessive sweating. We discussed how somatic anxiety can result from high leptin levels, and Marguerite decided to pursue a serum leptin test. As we saw with inflammation tests in chapter 4, leptin tests aren't generally performed clinically, so they are rarely covered by insurance, and most hospitals and laboratories aren't equipped for them. But Marguerite found a private provider and paid out of pocket for her test, which came back showing high leptin levels. Along with her symptoms, that was a strong sign to me that Marguerite was suffering from a condition called leptin resistance.

She changed her lifestyle over the following months to bring her leptin levels under control. Though she made a number of dietary changes, like emphasizing omega-3 fats over omega-6-rich vegetable oils (we'll talk more about different types of fats in part 2), the key for her was eliminating sugar. She had already cut down on obvious carbs, like bread and pasta, but she also had to be aware of the kinds of excess sugar that can lurk in sauces, salad dressings, and drinks. Once her diet was straightened out, Marguerite stopped hyperventilating, lost weight, and regained control over her life.

LEPTIN RESISTANCE

Why does leptin have such a seemingly contradictory relationship with anxiety? Is it really a Goldilocks situation where your brain needs precisely the right amount, with both too little and too much triggering anxiety? Not exactly.

Understanding these complicated relationships hinges on understanding the nuances of how hormones work in your body. For a hormone to be effective, your body requires two things: enough of the hormone to send the message *and* a properly functioning receptor to receive the message. That creates two possible ways in which the system can go awry. If your body isn't producing enough leptin, serum leptin levels stay low, and the lack of leptin in your brain can cause anxiety. But when you're overweight or obese, you naturally produce a lot of leptin—since leptin is manufactured and secreted by adipose tissue, an excess of adipose tissue means an excess of leptin. With too much leptin in your brain, your leptin receptors can malfunction and lose the ability to respond. Therefore, your brain can still be running a functional leptin deficit even as your endocrine system is continually pumping more into your brain, without being able to rectify the problem. Hence, your brain can still slip into anxiety even though your serum leptin levels are abnormally high.

This inability of your leptin receptors to function properly is called leptin resistance. It's similar to another major metabolic concern, insulin resistance, which we'll discuss in more detail in chapter 6, where the body loses the ability to respond to the hormone insulin, resulting in elevated blood sugar, which can lead to type 2 diabetes. In fact, leptin resistance and insulin resistance are so often found together that researchers speculate that the two may be causally linked.[23]

Leptin resistance puts both your body and mind in a difficult spot. Without being able to register the mediating presence of leptin, your brain doesn't know when to rein in your appetite or how to stay away from eating unhealthy foods that dial up more destruction, magnifying your anxiety in a variety of different ways. Treating leptin resistance is even more complicated than treating low leptin levels—after all, it's not a matter of increasing or decreasing your serum leptin; it's about retraining your body's leptin receptors to function properly.

Happily, it is possible to reset your leptin sensitivity through dedicated lifestyle changes, as we saw with Marguerite. Animal studies back this up: when obese rats who showed severe leptin resistance were put on a healthier diet, they fully regained leptin sensitivity.[24] Food choices for restoring leptin sensitivity are similar to those we discussed earlier for maintaining healthy leptin levels, such as the foods included in the Mediterranean diet. But research has shown that fighting leptin resistance is also about when and how much you eat. A variety of fasting and calorie-restrictive diets have been shown to be effective at helping to fight leptin resistance, but before trying any kind of radical diet, you should consult a professional, working to create an eating plan that is safe and healthy.[25]

If you are overweight and suspect you might be suffering from leptin resistance, the first thing to try is cutting out sugar. Several animal studies have established that a high-fructose diet causes leptin resistance in mice, regardless of the diet's fat content, and that when the mice were taken off the high-fructose diet, leptin sensitivity returned.[26] High-sugar meals have been shown to significantly increase leptin levels in overweight individuals, especially when that sugar comes from sweetened sodas.[27] Weaning yourself off sugar is a great first step toward resetting your relationship with leptin, improving your metabolic health, and lowering your anxiety.

AN APPETITE FOR FIGHTING ANXIETY

The difficulties of identifying, understanding, and treating leptin resistance are a good reminder that the factors that drive anxiety and struggles with your weight often have nothing to do with willpower. If your brain is unable to benefit from the calming effects of leptin on both your mood and appetite, that's not a moral failing or something to be ashamed of. It's simply a chemical issue in your body that can be rectified with knowledge and effort. That isn't made any easier by living in an era when unhealthy food is cheap and available at every turn, but with patience, proper planning, and fostering a love for whole, healthy foods, it's absolutely possible to take control of your diet and mental health.

In its management of fat stores and regulation of appetite, leptin has an important effect on your body's metabolism, the vastly complicated machinery that ensures you have the energy you need to live. Just as leptin dysfunction causes mental health symptoms, an off-kilter metabolism is one of the greatest risk factors for anxiety.

CHAPTER SIX

The Dangers of Metabolic Disruption

Javier was a fifty-six-year-old man who came to me with what I recognized as severe generalized anxiety. He was overwhelmed with increasing stressors at work, but switching to a less stressful career was out of the question because of the looming financial burden of funding his son's college education. He told me he had a constant fear of his life falling apart, of getting fired from work due to low performance, which would mean his son wouldn't be able to go to college and his wife would leave him. In talking through his issues, I could tell that these anxieties weren't based in reality—he played a stressful but crucial role at his job, and his wife and son loved him very much—but that didn't mean the anxiety wasn't causing very real damage to Javier, as well as taking a toll on his family. He was channeling his worry into arguing with his wife and being hard on his son in a way that was damaging the very relationships he was so concerned about preserving.

When we discussed his physical health, Javier admitted that he had been gaining weight, but amid his anxiety issues, he hadn't worried about it. Food sometimes felt like the only source of pleasure in his life, so he was willing to accept the added inches around his middle. He also told me that his weight gain had begun while taking an SSRI prescribed by his previous mental health professional, making him pack on pounds without alleviating his anxiety. I acknowledged that was one drawback of SSRIs and understood that he didn't want to rely on benzodiazepines for a short-term fix. That left us with therapy and a nutritional psychiatry treatment plan as our main ways to fight his anxiety.

He was willing to try therapy—though previous experiences with therapists hadn't yielded satisfying results—but he was more skeptical about undergoing dietary changes, at least until we did some blood tests. Javier's labs showed several signs of a disrupted metabolism. In addition to his problems with weight, he had an abnormal lipid profile. Most significantly, his blood sugar was off the charts. The tests meant that Javier had likely been suffering from metabolic syndrome for quite some time, which had developed into type 2 diabetes (T2D).

The diagnosis was a wake-up call that Javier had to make dietary changes to reduce his blood sugar. Gradually, as I explained the connection between metabolic health and mental health, he came around to the idea that his two conditions were linked and that eating healthier foods would also result in improvement to his anxiety. I told him how one study found that 40 percent of patients with diabetes suffered from elevated symptoms of anxiety, with 14 percent reaching the qualifications for a GAD diagnosis.[1] Another study found that clinically significant anxiety was 20 percent higher among Americans with diabetes, compared to healthy controls.[2] Further research has shown that less severe, subclinical anxiety is increased in diabetic populations as well.[3]

I was relieved that Javier was open to change, because the stakes were high. Anxiety makes metabolic recovery more difficult, and it is associated with more medical complications in T2D patients.[4]

I referred Javier to a cognitive behavioral therapist to help work on his negative thoughts and other psychological struggles. He felt more confident with a referral to a trusted practitioner than he had in the past when he was cold-calling clinics to book an appointment with a random therapist. We also designed a personalized nutritional psychiatry plan, slowly cutting back on less healthy habits and adding in healthy whole foods. We reduced snacking on so-called healthy protein bars that were laden with hidden added sugars, and we cleaned up his coffee routine, replacing sweet concoctions with simple drip coffee with unsweetened nut milk. We balanced his eating schedule, and since he was not much of a breakfast person, we tapped into the power of intermittent fasting.

Javier noticed changes within the first month, though it took longer for his metabolic profile to fully normalize. When his anxiety began to ease, he became even more engaged in his nutritional psychiatry treatment plan, and over six months, his blood sugar came back under control. He was once again able to enjoy time with his family and successfully sent his son to a great college.

WHAT IS METABOLISM?

To be alive, you need energy. You need energy to hug your pets and care for your children. You need energy to answer emails, to deal with coworkers, to clean the house. You need energy to exercise, to cook, to enjoy time with your friends. To complete all of life's challenges and experience all its joy, your body needs to be working at tip-top efficiency to convert the food you eat into vital energy.

We've already learned about the preliminary steps your body goes through to turn food into energy—for instance, in chapter 5 we learned about the role of leptin in managing your appetite and fat stores, and in chapters 2 and 3 we learned about how your gut breaks down food and fights off foreign invaders. After food is broken down, a series of chemical reactions takes place across your body, producing energy and delivering it to your cells to get you through your day. These processes are collectively called your metabolism.

You're probably most familiar with metabolism as it pertains to weight—according to the common usage of the term, someone with a "fast" metabolism can eat whatever they want without gaining weight, while someone with a "slow" metabolism gains weight even while eating less. The scientific truth is more complicated and nuanced than that. The medical term for the "speed" of your metabolism is basal metabolic rate and it's often overemphasized as a factor in weight loss, as well as oversimplifying the stunning complexity of the human body's energy-creation architecture. Your body is constantly performing a host of metabolic processes in an extraordinarily complicated web of chemical interactions that would make a biochemistry professor blush. While we won't get into the full complexity of how all these processes work, the two main types of metabolic reactions are catabolic reactions, which break down complex compounds into useful building blocks, and anabolic reactions, which build essential biological compounds like proteins from raw material.

As with any complicated system, much can go wrong with your metabolism. Errors in any part of the metabolic process, owing to either inborn defects or environmental stresses, can result in a metabolic disorder. For example, T2D is a malfunction of your body's ability to manage blood glucose (sugar). Glucose circulating in your blood is a primary source of your body's energy, and it's regulated by the hormone insulin, produced in the pancreas. Insulin helps your cells take in blood glucose, giving them power to perform the constant work of keeping you alive. But in T2D patients, either not enough insulin is being produced or your cells stop listening to the insulin, a condition called insulin resistance (as mentioned, similar to leptin resistance). Either way, if your cells aren't hearing insulin's orders to absorb glucose, that leaves the glucose circulating in your bloodstream. Initially, your pancreas might be able to mitigate the problem by pumping out more insulin, but without addressing the root cause, insulin resistance can worsen, and blood sugar can continue to rise. At intermediate blood sugar levels, patients are said to have prediabetes, and at high levels, they are diagnosed with full T2D. Excess blood sugar is toxic to your organs and tissues and can cause a variety of serious symptoms. Early on you might find yourself excessively thirsty and needing to urinate a lot, feeling tired and weak, or having blurred vision. Later, T2D can come with a host of life-threatening complications, like heart disease, blindness, circulatory issues, and nerve damage, leading to an increased risk to develop Alzheimer's disease or other types of dementia.

From this brief overview of T2D, you can see why it's considered a metabolic disease: it's caused by a fundamental flaw in your body's ability to process energy. But while T2D may be one of the most destructive metabolic diseases, it's far from the only one. With so many complexities surrounding energy processing, metabolic diseases have a wide variety of symptoms and causes.

Some metabolic disorders are genetic, caused by inherited errors in your body's energy-creation machinery. This could mean an inherited tendency toward high cholesterol ("familial hypercholesterolemia" in medical literature), or rarer and more severe conditions like Gaucher disease, Hunter's syndrome, and Tay-Sachs disease, which are often most prevalent in particular ethnic groups. Many of these serious conditions can be identified through genetic screening.

However, most metabolic disorders—including T2D—are brought on by lifestyle factors, especially poor diet and lack of exercise. Starting in the 1970s, as doctors began to understand the rapid increase and grave seriousness of these conditions, the term "metabolic syndrome" was coined to describe a constellation of factors that indicate an increased risk of serious health threats. Today, metabolic syndrome is defined as having any three of these five metabolic conditions:

- Excess abdominal fat

- Elevated triglycerides

- Low HDL, or so-called good cholesterol

- Elevated fasting blood sugar

- High blood pressure

Metabolic syndrome is associated with an increased risk of insulin resistance, prediabetes, and T2D; atherosclerosis, a hardening of the arteries that can lead to heart attack; and stroke. You'll recall some of those same life-threatening diseases from our discussion of chronic inflammation in chapter 4, and sure enough, inflammation appears to be tightly intertwined with metabolic syndrome, even though ongoing research is continuing to define these relationships more clearly.[5]

The serious implications of metabolic disease would be scary in any context. But they are downright terrifying when you consider how prevalent impaired metabolism is in today's United States. In examining data from 2009 to 2016, researchers came to the alarming conclusion that only 12.2 percent of Americans are achieving optimal metabolic health, and even in normal-weight adults, less than 33 percent were determined to be in peak metabolic condition.[6] That leaves about 88 percent of us with some impairment in our metabolic health! There has also been significant growth in the prevalence of metabolic syndrome in recent years, with 36.9 percent of Americans ticking at least three of the five diagnostic boxes.[7] And according to the most recent National Diabetes Statistical Report from the Centers for Disease Control and Prevention, an estimated 37.3 million people — 11.3 percent of the population — are living with diabetes, with a staggering 96 million people having prediabetes.[8]

While we are still learning much about the exact causes and

interactions of metabolic syndrome, T2D, and other metabolic disorders, their threat to health is undeniable. You'd be hard-pressed to find any doctor who doesn't recognize the gravity of these conditions and the importance of raising awareness and encouraging patients to take steps to prevent them. But as we've seen time and again, until the past few years, not much was understood about the grave implications that metabolic disease has for the brain. We are now learning that metabolic health *is* mental health, and vice versa.

Over the past several years, I have explored this on a deeper clinical level. In my opinion, the connection between metabolic conditions and mental health — which I call metabolic psychiatry — is the most significant link between the twin epidemics of poor physical and mental health. While that's sobering to think about, it also means that a healthy diet promoting strong metabolic health has the biggest potential for reducing anxiety.

ANXIETY AND METABOLIC HEALTH

I can understand why science has been slow to uncover the links between metabolism and anxiety. It's one thing to acknowledge how food and emotion can be tightly intertwined, because we have all experienced how our feelings respond to foods we eat. But after food is digested, metabolizing that food into raw energy seems like it would be as businesslike and impersonal as a hydroelectric turbine turning in a dam. Such a basic process shouldn't have the power to make you anxious, right? And surely *being* anxious wouldn't gum up the works of your body's energy-production machinery, would it?

Despite those reasonable assumptions, recent research indicates that metabolism and anxiety are indeed tightly connected. Metabolic profiles of anxious people are quite different from those of people who aren't anxious.[9] We already know about the associations between anxiety and T2D, but there are also links between anxiety and other metabolic indicators. Anxiety is associated with higher

LDL cholesterol and lower HDL cholesterol.[10] Anxiety's cousin depression has been linked to high HDL and triglycerides.[11] The association between cholesterol and anxiety is strong enough that there is even some evidence for using cholesterol-lowering statin drugs as an anxiety treatment.[12] These and other findings increasingly point to a strong link between anxiety and metabolism—but how can this be?

In chapter 1, we touched on the work of neuroscientist Lisa Feldman Barrett, who argues that the brain did not evolve for thinking or feeling. Rather, our brains evolved to ensure that we have sufficient resources to grow, survive, and reproduce. The most important resource for all these biological imperatives is *energy*, and as we know, the body derives that energy from food via metabolism. In that sense, in its quest to set you up to thrive, one of the brain's main functions is to act as a metabolic adjuster, ensuring that your metabolism is providing the energy you need to be productive and protect yourself from threat and danger. While you may not be consciously aware of it, your brain is pulling every possible lever to ensure that you have the energy you need—including manipulating your mood.

To manage your metabolism, your brain must communicate with the ANS, the immune system, and the endocrine system (which secretes hormones like insulin). Just as we saw in our study of leptin in chapter 5, many parts of the brain that connect with the systems that control metabolism are the same ones that are central to anxiety—especially the amygdala and hippocampus. Yes, metabolism and emotions are both generated from the same places in the brain. To me this was a mind-blowing revelation.

This overlap of metabolism and mental health fits in with Barrett's theory that emotions are the result of the brain preparing for the future. Your brain is constantly scanning your body's metabolic state and triggering changes in your mood and behavior to maintain the best path forward. In recent scientific studies, researchers have uncovered how the brain can use emotions to control energy balance, finding that hunger can lead to a suppression of fear to encourage you to seek out food, ignoring the risk of danger. On the other hand, when you are overweight or obese, your brain can turn your fear response back up, discouraging you from taking unnecessary risks to acquire more food.[13] In other words, there is a possible evolutionary underpinning for the idea that being overweight can lead to anxiety—your brain reads excess weight as a sign that it needs to scare you into being more risk-averse when gathering food.

Of course, in the modern world, gathering food is not risky at all—the ability to go to the supermarket or a fast-food restaurant and safely obtain an unlimited supply of sustenance means we're at far more risk of eating too much than of eating too little. So instead of our anxiety scaring us into diminishing our fat stores, we keep eating unhealthy food and gaining weight, which further skews our metabolism, which leads to more anxiety. It's yet another vicious cycle that can be disrupted only by making healthier food choices.

ANOTHER TWO-WAY STREET

As we've seen at nearly every point in this book, it's difficult to sort out the cause and effect of anxiety and metabolism, because both feed on each other. There's ample evidence that metabolic disease worsens anxiety, and that anxiety worsens metabolic disease. In Javier's case, I suspect there was a bit of both. His diet issues were at the root of both his mental health struggles and his high blood sugar, each worsening the other until we addressed the underlying problem. Many studies have turned up similar findings, with anxiety appearing as comorbid with metabolic syndrome,[14] obesity,[15] and more specific metabolic conditions like nonalcoholic fatty liver disease.[16]

There are clear examples of metabolic processes leading to anxiety. For example, certain metabolism byproducts are called reactive oxygen species, which, despite the misleading name, are not a species of organism but highly reactive and toxic oxygen compounds. You may have heard of oxidative stress, caused by an overproduction of reactive oxygen species, which is harmful to cells. Oxidative stress is understood to be a precursor to metabolic diseases like diabetes, as well as cancer and cardiovascular disease. Sure enough, research has also shown that oxidative stress is a driver of anxiety.[17] The story gets even more complicated, but I won't spend more time going into the biochemistry of other alterations in energy balance such as mitochondrial regulation, glutamine metabolism, and neurotransmission, all of which have also been found to promote anxiety.

On the other side of cause and effect, while anxiety is far from the sole cause of metabolic disorders—there are certainly people with disrupted metabolisms who don't experience mental health symptoms at all—there are clear indications that consistent stress and anxiety can be a catalyst for future metabolic issues. For instance, as we learned in chapter 5 when discussing leptin, anxiety can lead to overeating and choosing unhealthy foods, which leads to increased weight and therefore metabolic risk. Chronic stress has been shown to cause an increase in visceral fat (fat that concentrates around your organs, rather than under the surface of your skin), which has been identified as a strong risk factor for metabolic disease.

There are even indications that early-life stress can have implications for your risk of contracting metabolic disease later in life. Mothers who undergo significant stress during pregnancy are more likely to have babies with low birth weight, which is somewhat paradoxically correlated with an increased likelihood to suffer from obesity, hypertension, and diabetes later in life. Similar results have been found in children who undergo significant stresses later in childhood. A fascinating study focused on the Helsinki Birth Cohort, a group of Finnish participants who, as children, were separated from their parents when evacuated to other countries during

World War II. Later in life they were more likely to develop cardiovascular disease and T2D.[18]

METABOLITES

Thus far, we have been focusing on the correlation between anxiety and major metabolic markers that are regularly tested for in a clinical setting—weight, blood sugar, cholesterol, triglycerides, and blood pressure are points of emphasis at your yearly physical. But researchers are also finding connections between anxiety and metabolism through the study of less heralded compounds called metabolites. We saw the effect of metabolites produced by your gut bacteria when discussing neurotransmitter synthesis in chapter 2, but your own metabolic processes produce metabolites as well. Studying metabolites produced by your gut bacteria and your body can shed light on complicated metabolic diseases that are otherwise difficult to pin down. The sum total of metabolites in a sample is called the metabolome (echoing our old friend the microbiome), and this emerging field of study is called metabolomics.

Metabolomics has potential as a diagnostic tool. Given how many granular differences there are among different individuals' metabolomes, in the future, they are potentially useful in identifying and diagnosing conditions, including mental health conditions. For example, we know that depression and anxiety often occur together and can sometimes be so interrelated that it is difficult to tell them apart. Though the field is far from being fully developed, metabolomics offers one possible path toward being able to differentiate the two conditions, via blood test. A 2021 study of individuals who were suffering from anxiety, those suffering from depression, those suffering from both conditions at once, and healthy controls found that all four groups had slightly different metabolomes, raising the possibility that we might be able to diagnose these conditions through metabolic testing in the future.[19]

There are also indications that metabolites aren't just markers of anxiety but are actually causing or contributing to anxiety themselves. For example, in 2022, researchers at Caltech observed that when a gut-derived metabolite called 4EPS was present in the brains of lab mice, it triggered anxious behavior. While much more research is needed to implicate 4EPS specifically in human anxiety, this is a valuable sign of the gut's role in anxiety, and that abnormal metabolites can contribute to anxious states.[20]

As with 4EPS, many metabolites and their precursors are produced in the gut, with a crucial assist from your microbiome. Based on signaling from metabolites, cells in your gut mucosa make and release a variety of hormones that have an effect on insulin sensitivity, glucose tolerance, and other metabolic processes.[21] Furthermore, managing the makeup of your microbiome through diet has been shown to have an effect on metabolic profile, and there is great potential for using gut health to treat metabolic conditions.[22]

As metabolomics continues to make strides, I'm excited to see new ways in which metabolites shed light on both the diagnosis and treatment of anxiety, to gain a greater understanding of the connections between metabolic health and gut health.

METABOLIZING ANXIETY

Though much of the research surrounding metabolism and anxiety is still in early stages, I want to emphasize that I have seen these associations playing out in very real ways many times in my clinic. In addition to Javier, I have treated a thirty-year-old woman named Tyra, whose anxiety was connected to the thyroid condition Graves' disease, which has long been known to be a driver of mental distress.[23] I treated Angie, a forty-year-old whose lack of time to prepare healthy food was wreaking havoc on her weight as her metabolism slowed with age — something that is scientifically proven to happen to us all.[24] She was suffering from vicious anxiety and self-hatred until we normalized her cholesterol by instituting a strict exercise regimen and replacing some of her unhealthy choices with healthier ones. I treated Peng Shui, a new mother who thought she was suffering from postpartum anxiety but was actually experiencing an interaction between cholesterol levels and anxiety that has been shown to affect women who have recently given birth.[25]

While the future might hold the possibility of going to a metabolomics clinic to receive a complete workup that lays out an individualized treatment plan, for now the absolute best thing you can do to ensure your mental and metabolic health is to eat a diet full of metabolically healthy food, maintain weight control, and keep levels of cholesterol, triglycerides, and blood sugar in an optimal range.

Now that we are armed with knowledge gleaned from the latest research about the connections between diet and anxiety, it's time to dive into specifics on how to translate this knowledge into an actionable plan for eating a gut- and brain-healthy diet that will keep you anxiety-free.

That means it's time to turn our attention to my favorite subject: food.

PART II: THE SOLUTION

CHAPTER SEVEN

Macronutrients

Ahanu, forty years old, had recently been promoted to senior sales leader at a Fortune 500 company. His new role was exciting but stressful, involving a vast amount of air travel across the globe and a breakneck schedule that often meant long hours every day of the week. While he had steeled himself for pressure and hard work, Ahanu hadn't expected mounting symptoms of anxiety. He was finding himself on the brink of panic attacks during his frequent travel, which he had never experienced before. Even routine interactions at work, like chatting with colleagues in the break room, greeting his boss, and simply deciding how to dress for work, were causing him to spend hours obsessing about what he said and how he acted, costing him sleep and leaving him feeling constantly jumpy and irritable.

When Ahanu came to my clinic for a consultation, we discussed the difficulties of adjusting to the stress and pressure of his new job and talked about the possibility that imposter syndrome was rearing its head. And, of course, we evaluated his diet. Ahanu came from Native American roots and was the first in his family to work in the corporate world. He grew up on his family's farm and was used to eating a traditional diet based mostly on low-fat, high-protein, complex carbohydrate–based foods like heirloom varieties of corn, field beans, squash, root crops, and native berries.

Early in his career, Ahanu had largely maintained his traditional diet as a way to stay connected to his upbringing and heritage — and simply because it was a delicious and familiar way to sustain himself. But as his star rose in the company, it was harder to make the time to shop and cook. When he was on the road, he was relying on airport pastries and lavish client dinners designed to be decadent and impressive rather than nourishing. When he was home with the kids, he was tired and wanted to treat them, so they would end up going out for pizza and fast-food meals rather than cooking. I explained to Ahanu that the macronutrients in his diet had gotten twisted around. Instead of eating a largely plant-based diet full of fiber-rich beans and low-glycemic-index carbs from locally grown vegetables, he was eating doughnuts and porterhouse drenched in butter.

I started Ahanu on an SSRI to help ease his anxiety, but I also encouraged him to find ways to get back to his old eating patterns. We talked about how he could make preparing traditional meals a fun activity to do with his family when he was between trips, as well as how to prepare food in advance that he could take with him during his travels. I encouraged a plant-rich diet, adding back the beans and root vegetables he grew up with, as well as exploring some new styles of cooking. Easy meals became his go-to dinners for the family and gave him healthy leftovers for lunch the next day — for instance, oven-baked salmon with my Miso-Infused Cipollini Onions and Green Beans (page 259). He also made a five-bean stew — loaded with vegetables — in the crockpot and served it with a side of seasoned wild rice. When he traveled, he ate large salads with the dressing on the side. While client meals were part of the job, he decided he would nudge plans out of fancier fine-dining options (with few to no calming dishes) and toward healthier wow-factor meals like sushi. And when that wasn't possible, he opted for baked or grilled fish, rather than an anxiety-inducing meal.

Before long, Ahanu told me that he was feeling more at ease in his new role, staying focused on his professional goals. Returning to his traditional diet also deepened his bond with his family and helped him reconnect with his heritage. Changing the biggest components of his diet — macronutrients — changed his life.

In this chapter, we'll study the ways in which fat, carbohydrates, and protein can exacerbate or alleviate anxiety.

WHAT ARE MACRONUTRIENTS?

Macronutrients — fat, carbohydrates, and protein — are the biggest components of the food we eat. Most healthy diets consist of some proportion of all three. Of course, the devil is in the details. What is the right balance? What are the best and worst sources of each? And how do they factor into anxiety?

Those questions don't always have easy answers, and changing attitudes about macronutrients can lead to shifting sands of advice. Take fat, for example. Starting in the late 1940s, when much of the foundation of modern nutritional thought was forming, researchers found associations between high-fat diets and high cholesterol, a metabolic risk factor that was correlated with a greater risk of heart disease. Thus, a low-fat diet was assumed to lower cholesterol and lead to better heart health. At first, low-fat diets were recommended only for those at risk of heart disease, but through the fifties and sixties, they became a prescription for everyone. In the eighties and nineties, a fully-fledged lifestyle blossomed that promoted low-fat diets not only for heart health but also weight loss. Doctors, governments, and public sentiment agreed that fat consumption should be as low as possible, and that the healthiest fat to consume was vegetable oil. Margarine replaced butter. Chicken — especially boneless, skinless chicken breasts — replaced fattier meats. Skim milk was king. Brands labeled every possible food as "low-fat" and "heart-healthy," even if they were packed with calories and sugar.[1]

In the 2000s, the pendulum started to swing the other way. After years of certainty that fat was at the root of bad health and excess weight, negative attention turned to a different macronutrient: carbohydrates. While low-carb diets had been used for weight loss since the nineteenth century, they rose to new prominence as wave after wave of trendy diets that cut carbs started to take over the popular health consciousness.[2] Today, diets recommending an eighties- or nineties-style low-fat approach are much less common, but there are still plenty of diets predicated on low carb intake, including the popular ketogenic diet, which we will discuss in chapter 11.

Who was right, the anti-fat crusaders or the anti-carb crusaders? Both of them. And neither of them. Despite what some diet evangelists will tell you, no one macronutrient should be totally ostracized, and there isn't a definitive balance of macronutrients that is better than all others. Consider how diets heavy in different macronutrients affect conditions like T2D, which has a strong correlation with anxiety. The traditional approach to treating T2D through diet is to eat a low-fat, low-calorie diet in order to normalize blood sugar and other metabolic indicators—a similar line of thinking to the original low-fat recommendations from the fifties. But recently, low-carb diets like the ketogenic diet have gained prominence in treating T2D and have shown that they can be even more effective, reducing the need for diabetic medications and even forcing T2D into remission.[3] However, recent research showed that a high-starch, plant-based diet from the BROAD study—which has a very different macronutrient makeup than a keto diet—was extremely effective at helping study participants with T2D lose weight and improve cholesterol and other metabolic risk factors.[4] Rather than insisting that there must be a single optimal dietary treatment for T2D, it's better to recognize that several different approaches can be effective and that methods can be tailored to patient preference and situation. This is part of a broader movement to a much more personalized form of medicine in all medical specialties, but it's particularly important when considering dietary interventions.

There are also many ways in which the balance of macronutrients in your diet can improve or worsen anxiety directly. Much of the low-fat-versus-low-carb debate happened before we really understood the connection between food and mental health, but with our current knowledge, we are beginning to see that prioritizing one macronutrient over the others can risk worsening anxiety. For example, a low-fat diet might leave you short of valuable omega-3 fatty acids, which are hugely important in fighting anxiety. A low-carb diet might make it hard to get proper amounts of dietary fiber, which plays a crucial role in regulating the gut microbiome. A low-protein diet (or one that doesn't include a diverse selection of proteins) could result in a lack of essential amino acids like tryptophan.

In other words, when making recommendations for my patients, I try to keep from getting wrapped up in absolutes — there is no one type of macronutrient that can be eliminated to cure anxiety. But just because I don't think fat or carbs are an all-or-nothing proposition, that doesn't mean that macronutrient balance and quality don't matter. I am glad we have left behind the era of demonizing all fat, but I certainly acknowledge the importance of reducing or eliminating unhealthy fats, as well as promoting healthy fats. The same is true of carbs. While a low-carb lifestyle isn't a guaranteed ticket to a calm mind, there are certain types of carbs that should be avoided and others prioritized. When it comes to protein, proponents of a vegan diet are vocal about avoiding animal protein at all costs, while ardent meat eaters will claim that you can never be truly healthy on a totally plant-based diet. In reality, it's possible to reduce anxiety as a vegan or a meat eater, as long as you make conscious, informed choices about the proteins you eat.

Spending time on social media, watching morning shows, and even discussing food with your friends and family can quickly induce anxiety as you encounter strong, often conflicting opinions. But by understanding macronutrients, you'll be better equipped to determine the best ways to eat for your brain and body — and your anxiety.

FATS

The negative connotations surrounding the word "fat" tend to cloud discussions about the important role of fat in your body and diet. Between the demonization of dietary fat in the late twentieth century and harmful body standards that encourage burning fat at all costs, it's easy to see why it is such a loaded term. But fat is necessary for a healthy life. In chapter 5, we learned how your adipose tissue is actually an advanced endocrine organ that helps manage your body's long-term energy needs. Fat is also a crucial part of your diet, providing a great source of energy, helping you dissolve and absorb nutrients, and supplying you with essential fatty acids that your body can't make on its own. Essential fatty acids are particularly important for mental health, since your brain is nearly 60 percent fat and relies on a steady supply of dietary fats to maintain proper function.[5]

Of course, not all fats are created equal. Let's break down the different kinds of fats and learn which ones to prioritize and which to avoid as you make antianxiety eating choices.

Unsaturated Fats

There are two main types of unsaturated fats, monounsaturated fats (made up of monounsaturated fatty acids, or MUFAs) and polyunsaturated fats (made up of polyunsaturated fatty acids, or PUFAs). The difference between the two has to do with their chemical structure, with "mono" and "poly" referring to the number of double bonds in their fatty acid chains. An easy way to distinguish unsaturated fats from saturated fats is that unsaturated fats are nearly always liquid at room temperature, whereas saturated fats are solid at room temperature (though certain unsaturated fats, like margarine and vegetable shortening, undergo processing that allows them to be solid at room temperature). MUFAs and PUFAs are generally regarded as healthier than their saturated cousins, but it's worth considering the details before assuming that all unsaturated fats are perfectly healthy with no danger of increasing anxiety.

MUFAs make up the bulk of fats in olive oil, avocados, most nuts, and some cooking oils. MUFAs are nearly always recognized as being healthy, particularly olive oil and avocado oil. Olive oil is the primary cooking fat of Mediterranean cultures, whose low rates of heart disease inspired nutritionists worldwide to create and recommend the Mediterranean diet, which has also been shown to fight depression and anxiety.[6] Avocado oil has many of the same benefits as olive oil, while being better for high-temperature cooking like sautéing and stir-frying.

There are a myriad of studies that show that high-MUFA diets promote gut health,[7] fight inflammation,[8] and lead to decreased metabolic risk factors[9] as well as lower levels of anxiety.[10] Not all MUFAs should be eaten in unlimited quantities—for instance, while certain cooking oils like canola and peanut oil contain MUFAs, they tend to be used in deep-frying, which is likely to lead to consuming a ton of calories' worth of refined carbs. While I suggest my patients limit these cooking oils, I certainly encourage them to eat healthy fats from olive oil, avocados and avocado oil, nuts, and seeds.

PUFAs have two important subsets. Omega-6 PUFAs include most vegetable cooking oils found in processed foods—corn oil, sunflower oil, and safflower oil are all types of PUFAs. Like MUFAs, these fats are regarded as relatively healthy in very small quantities, though it's important to acknowledge that they are often a major component of unhealthy foods. No fat is healthy when combined in large amounts with high-glycemic-load carbohydrates that practically beg you to stuff yourself with them. In other words, French fries aren't healthy. While evidence is somewhat mixed, there are signs that omega-6 PUFAs have been linked to anxiety and depression,[11] and they can be pro-inflammatory,[12] so I generally encourage my patients to limit them, especially in fried, processed, and packaged foods.

On the other hand, omega-3 PUFAs are some of the most

important fats for mental health. There are three main types of omega-3 fatty acids: EPA and DHA, which are found in fatty fish like salmon, and ALA, which largely comes from plant sources like seeds, nuts, seaweed, and other types of algae. DHA is particularly crucial in brain development, and babies who don't get enough DHA can have a variety of troubles as their brains grow. Later in life, omega-3s have powerful anti-inflammatory properties; they are a crucial tool in fighting anxiety-causing neuroinflammation, which we discussed in chapter 4.[13] While much of the research surrounding omega-3s' effect on mental health is centered around depression and neurodegenerative diseases, there is growing evidence that omega-3s directly reduce anxiety as well.[14]

Given our understanding of the importance of omega-3s, omega-3 supplements are available that give you a certain ratio of EPA, DHA, and ALA as a pill or capsule. While I don't categorically object to supplements, it's worth acknowledging that in many studies, dietary sources of omega-3s yielded better results than supplements.[15] Additionally, no one enjoys choking down a large capsule of fish oil, but many enjoy eating a well-cooked piece of salmon. For my anxious patients who don't object to eating fish for other reasons, I heartily recommend that they take the time to learn to cook salmon in order to capitalize on the best source of EPA and DHA. Those who prefer a plant-based diet can eat flaxseeds, chia seeds, and walnuts for ALA, and EPA and DHA are also available via vegan algal oil supplements.

One important way to think about your PUFA intake is to try to eat a proper ratio of omega-6 fats to omega-3 fats. Given how much vegetable oil we consume compared to how little fish we consume, it can be very easy to skew this ratio—with the average American consuming in the vicinity of 15 to 1 omega-6s to omega-3s, according to some estimates. Studies have found that balancing out that ratio, ideally to lower than 5 to 1, yields many health benefits, largely resulting from a reduction in inflammatory conditions.[16] Improving this ratio has also been shown to directly decrease anxiety.[17] Of course, it's not always practical or even possible to determine the exact amount of omega-6s and omega-3s in your diet, so I simply encourage patients to try to eat fewer omega-6 fats and more omega-3 fats.

Saturated Fats

When you think of fatty foods, your mind might drift to the smell of sizzling bacon or the taste of melted butter. These are types of saturated fat, which is largely derived from animal sources. Unlike MUFAs and PUFAs, saturated fat is usually solid at room temperature — the bacon grease and melted butter will turn back into solids as they cool. The few plant sources of saturated fat, like coconut and palm kernel oil, are also solid or semisolid at room temperature.

Saturated fats have a reputation for being unhealthy, and as with all foods, I certainly recommend that my patients moderate their intake of them. Saturated fat has traditionally been considered a factor in heart health, and for years guidance has been to eat as little as possible in order to reduce risk of heart attack and other cardiovascular conditions. High cholesterol due to a diet rich in saturated fat is also one of the pillars of metabolic syndrome, which we learned in chapter 6 is a risk factor for metabolic conditions like T2D. And sure enough, there have been studies linking consumption of saturated fat to increased anxiety,[18] as well as anxiety-producing conditions like neuroinflammation.[19]

However, saturated fats are currently one of the biggest areas of conflict in the study of nutrition. After years of recommending little to no saturated fat intake, studies are now suggesting that saturated fats may not be as harmful as we thought. In a landmark study from 2020, the *Journal of the American College of Cardiology* found that saturated fat from whole-fat dairy, unprocessed meat, and dark chocolate do not have an effect on heart-disease risk and can actually be protective against conditions like stroke.[20] While more research is needed on what these findings mean for mental health conditions like anxiety, it's becoming clear that saturated fats have also been overly vilified in the past. Upon reviewing the most recent literature on saturated fats, I've embraced recommending sensible amounts of full-fat dairy, butter, and some cuts of ethically farmed beef. These foods are quite rich in protein as well as vitamins and minerals, so changes in saturated fat guidelines make them worthy additions to your diet, at least in moderation.

Trans Fats

While new scientific research has led to an improvement in saturated fat's reputation, that is very much *not* the case for trans fats. Though small amounts of trans fats do occur in natural sources, they're largely man-made through a process called hydrogenation. Ironically, trans fats proliferated during the low-fat craze of the second half of the twentieth century—given the bad reputation of saturated fats, snack makers looked for a non-saturated fat that was still solid at room temperature. The solution was partially hydrogenated oil, which is a major source of trans fats. It began to appear in butter substitutes like margarine, chips, cakes, cookies, and almost every form of processed snack food.

What was originally pitched as a healthier alternative to saturated fat turned out to be just the opposite. Trans fats have been implicated in increased risk of heart disease, T2D, obesity, and even cancer.[21] Many of these ill effects are likely related to its pro-inflammatory tendencies, as trans fats contribute to chronic systemic inflammation.[22] Unsurprisingly, trans fats have been directly linked to higher levels of anxiety in both animal[23] and human studies.[24]

During the 2000s, many governments, including the US government, took measures to ban trans fats, which has helped reduce the risk of exposure. However, due to lobbying from the processed-food industry and the slow timeline of advancing legislation, the ban was not actually enacted until 2018, with products produced before the ban allowed to stay on the market until 2020. Even in 2022, it's possible for older processed foods to contain high levels of trans fats, so that's another reason I always encourage patients to limit any processed, packaged junk food and fried food from restaurants.

As knowledge about the dangers of trans fats grew, producers of cooking fats like vegetable shortening moved to fully hydrogenated oils, which yield a similar product without the trans fats. However, given how heavily processed shortening is—and given that it is usually used in sweets and processed snacks—I still recommend avoiding it.

CARBOHYDRATES

When you think of carbohydrates, your mind probably jumps to starches: bread, rice, pasta, potatoes, and other dietary staples. Those are certainly major sources of carbs in traditional diets around the world. But sugar is the simplest form of carb, and it makes up a huge part of the caloric load in many modern diets, especially the standard American diet. More complex carbs come from fruits like apples, vegetables like broccoli, and legumes like lentils. When you think about cutting carbs, are you committing to eliminating broccoli and lentils? I doubt it. That's why, amid volleys of arguments from different factions in the carb wars, I try to keep a level-headed approach when advising my patients. Treating carbs as a monolithic, universally harmful food group just isn't useful, and I think it's time for a more sensible approach.

Most research and discourse surrounding carbs concerns improving metabolic health. But remember, metabolic health *is* mental health. As we'll see, the recommendations about carb consumption that improve metabolic health will improve anxiety, too.

Carb Quality and Glycemic Index

Just as we saw with fats, it's all about eating *quality* carbs. The idea that your body processes every carbohydrate the same way simply is not true. There is ample evidence that different types of carbs have different metabolic effects on your body. Some are more energy efficient than others, providing your body with more power for the amount you consume. Some are pro-inflammatory and come with greater risks of the kinds of metabolic health factors we discussed in chapter 6. Others bring along increased levels of important nutritional components like dietary fiber.

I won't get too deep into the nutritional chemistry that determines carb quality, but I do want to highlight an important concept that helps determine which carbs to eat and which to avoid. The glycemic index (GI) is a 100-point scale that measures how quickly different carbohydrates raise your blood sugar — in other words, how long it takes for the food you eat to turn into energy in your bloodstream. In most cases, a lower score is better for you, because it means less of a spike in blood sugar, which can stress your metabolism and lead to metabolic conditions that are risk factors for anxiety.

Pure glucose sets the top of the range with a glycemic index of 100, while more complex carbs that take longer to digest have lower scores. High glycemic index foods (GI scores of 70 and above) include white bread, white rice, peeled potatoes, and many processed breakfast cereals. Medium glycemic index foods (GI scores of 56–69) include whole wheat bread, basmati rice, unpeeled potatoes, and certain fruits like bananas and grapes. Low glycemic index foods (GI scores of 55 or less) include intact grains like oats and brown rice, mushrooms, and fruits like peaches and berries.

Diets heavy in high-GI carbs have been correlated with higher rates of anxiety in both animal and observational human studies[25] as well as in case studies of specific patients.[26] High-GI diets have also been found to be risk factors for depression,[27] lead to a higher concentration of inflammatory markers,[28] and contribute to poor metabolic health[29] — a familiar lineup of anxiety comorbidities. So even if you don't have any interest in seriously limiting carbs, I encourage replacing processed foods and other high-GI carbs with low-GI carbs. Instead of a processed breakfast cereal, have a bowl of steel-cut oats with berries. Instead of potatoes, choose sweet potatoes or, even better, carrots or a more adventurous root vegetable like taro. Instead of a sugary dessert, go for an apple, orange, or banana.

In recent years, some of my patients who struggle with blood sugar have used continuous glucose monitors, devices that track blood glucose levels at all times, allowing you to see exactly how different foods affect your blood sugar. Though their results generally track with conventional wisdom on glycemic index, I've also come across some surprising results, where blood sugar spikes more or less dramatically than I would expect in relation to different foods. My takeaway from this clinical data is that we are each unique, and each person's response to a certain food may differ. This is another sign that we need personalized medicine moving forward.

Fiber Is Your Friend

Another major plus for foods rich in low-GI carbohydrates is that they tend to be higher in dietary fiber, which is a crucial part of an anxiety-lowering diet. Dietary fiber is not actually a carb itself, but its main sources are carb-rich foods like fruits, vegetables, legumes, and whole grains. Fiber plays a unique role in nutrition because it's a nutrient that we can't actually digest and absorb into our bodies. Even though our bodies can't turn fiber into energy, it still helps to control appetite, slow digestion, ease the passage of waste, and promote a healthy gut microbiome.

In recent research, dietary fiber has emerged as one of the most important factors in fighting anxiety with food. For instance, in a 2021 study from Iran, high-fiber diets were significantly correlated with lower levels of anxiety.[30] Furthermore, fiber has been shown to be a bulwark against inflammation and depression as well.[31] And fiber has long been known to lead to better metabolic health indicators like cholesterol levels.[32]

These positive effects of fiber are partially attributable to its importance to gut health. Remember from chapter 2 that different gut microbiota thrive on different types of substances in your gut. Foods that provide nourishment for bacteria are called prebiotics, and fiber is one of the most advantageous types of prebiotic, promoting helpful strains of bacteria, discouraging toxic strains, increasing absorption of minerals, and improving gut permeability and immune response.[33] Furthermore, recent evidence suggests that the bacteria that produce important metabolism-regulating substances like SCFAs thrive on the dietary fiber passing through your gut.[34] In other words, ample fiber in your diet means a greater concentration of good bacteria, which leads to good gut health, which in turn results in good metabolic health and less anxiety.

Given the prevalence of processed carbs in the modern US diet, it's quite common to fall short of the proper amount of fiber in your diet—most adults need at least 25–35 grams of fiber per day, but the typical American diet includes only about 15 grams per day.[35] Getting enough fiber can be particularly difficult on a low-carb diet, which focuses on fats and proteins from animal and seafood sources that have little to no fiber content. Fiber comes from plants, especially whole grains, fruits, nuts, beans, lentils, and leafy greens. While you can supplement your diet with fiber from natural sources like psyllium husk (the key ingredient in fiber mixes sold under brands like Metamucil), foods rich in fiber are healthy in so many ways that I heartily encourage you to try to get as much fiber as you can from whole foods first.

Sugar (and Artificial Sweeteners)

We've seen several patients in the book whose anxiety was worsened by excess sugar in their diet. That checks out with what we know about high-GI carbs promoting anxiety, since sugars are among the highest GI foods, providing quick raw energy without delivering much else in the way of nutrition. We all know the feeling of the "sugar rush," where you get a burst of energy after eating something sweet, followed quickly by the "sugar crash," where your energy collapses. That can lead to eating more sugar to regain the high, which turns into a cycle of bad diet choices and leads to anxiety.

A large cross-sectional study from France found that nondiabetic individuals under forty-five with anxiety ate more sugar than those without anxiety.[36] Sugar consumption has also been correlated with depression[37] and is one of the primary drivers of bad metabolic health.[38] Eating a lot of sugar can mean disruptions in gut health as well, leading to a welcoming environment for pro-inflammatory bacteria while discouraging the anti-inflammatory bacteria that help maintain the integrity of your gut mucosa.[39] If you haven't noticed, these effects are the polar opposite of what we just saw with dietary fiber. In all the ways dietary fiber helps your physical health and fights anxiety, sugar harms your physical health and feeds anxiety.

Unfortunately, we just don't *crave* dietary fiber the same way we crave sugar. I'm sure you've heard people say they have a "sugar addiction" in a joking manner, but the similarities between compulsive sugar consumption and drug addiction are quite real. The brain pathways that sugar activates are similar to those activated by drugs like opioids.[40] The sweet tooth is a powerful thing, and I believe that's a big reason why anxiety is so rampant.

Of course, while sugar's role in causing anxiety is only recently becoming understood, it hasn't been a secret that sugar is bad for your health. That has driven people to try to satisfy their sweet tooth while avoiding the ill effects of sugar, turning to artificial sweeteners like sucralose (Splenda) and aspartame (sold under the brands NutraSweet and Equal, and used in many diet sodas such as Diet Coke). In July 2023, aspartame was listed as a possible carcinogen to humans by the WHO, the International Agency for Research on Cancer (IARC), and the Joint Expert Committee on Food Additives (JECFA). While the IARC cited limited evidence, this is still worth noting.[41] Unfortunately, studies have found that artificial sweeteners are not quite as magical as they might appear, since they promote gut dysbiosis by providing bad gut bacteria with a feast — remember Tilo, whom we met in chapter 2? Aspartame in particular has been linked with anxiety symptoms in both animal studies[42] and human studies,[43] but I discourage artificial sweeteners across the board. If you absolutely cannot live without them, erythritol is a natural sweetener that cannot be digested by you or your gut bacteria, so it is less likely to cause anxiety and metabolic dysfunction.[44] Another new option is allulose, a compound that naturally occurs in certain fruits. While there hasn't yet been any research on its role in anxiety, research into its effects on metabolic health has looked promising, so it may be worth trying in moderation.

Gluten

A particularly contentious subset of the carb wars is the potentially harmful effects of gluten, a protein found in several grains, most importantly wheat. As evidenced by the explosion of gluten-free diets, gluten-free bakeries, and aggressive food labeling to announce products as gluten-free (whether they could reasonably contain gluten or not—for example, I've even seen "gluten-free" water!), there has been a growing movement toward discouraging gluten. It's important to note that gluten is not harmful to everyone. Unlike sugar and trans fats, it is not inherently bad for you. However, a small percentage of people react poorly to gluten in a very real way, and the prevalence of these negative reactions has increased dramatically over the past few decades. Scientists attribute this increase in gluten intolerance to changes in the wheat supply. Today's wheat has been hybridized and modified until it is quite different from the original ancient grain. Industrial farming, designed to be as cheap and efficient as possible while yielding the largest harvests possible, has truly harmed the quality of our grains, which has changed the ways our body reacts to them.[45]

Gluten intolerance is most clearly seen in sufferers of celiac disease. Celiac is a chronic autoimmune disease that causes gluten to trigger an immune response in your gut, damaging parts of your gut mucosa. The result is a host of symptoms, including fatigue, diarrhea, and decreased absorption of crucial nutrients. Remembering what we know about the role of the immune system in the gut mucosa from chapter 3, it's unsurprising that celiac has also been linked to anxiety. Among many individual studies showing this association, a 2020 review of thirty-seven studies found that celiac comes with an increased chance of anxiety, as well as other mental health conditions like depression and ADHD.[46] Since celiac is treated by avoiding gluten, going gluten-free may very well help alleviate anxiety, too. Still, celiac presents in only about 1 percent of the population—fairly high for a chronic condition, but still not super common.

Complicating matters is a more prevalent but less well understood condition called gluten sensitivity, which is estimated to affect six times more people than celiac. Gluten sensitivity is not necessarily a precursor or a mild case of celiac but is rooted in a different kind of immune response. While there is much more to understand about gluten sensitivity, some studies have tied it to anxiety.[47]

If you are suffering from anxiety and feel you are sensitive to gluten—for instance, if you notice bloating, gas, or other gastrointestinal distress after eating food made from wheat—going gluten-free could help improve your anxiety even if you test negative for celiac. But unless you have a strong reason to believe gluten could be the culprit, I always recommend focusing on carb quality before you worry too much about gluten specifically. And since issues with gluten are tied to industrial farming, the source of gluten is also key: a slice of processed store-bought bread is different from an artisanal loaf of sourdough made from heritage grains and a fermented starter.

PROTEIN

Compared to the other two macronutrients, protein is less controversial. There are arguments over which protein sources are best, but it's widely agreed that protein is important. Low-protein diets do exist, but they are used only in rare cases, for instance, when treating kidney and liver disease. In other words, I'm not concerned about a low-protein diet catching on as the next major shift in macronutrient thought.

Perhaps because of its universal acceptance as an important dietary component, there's not a wide body of research on how protein affects anxiety. There is evidence that protein malnourishment can promote anxiety — for example, a 2020 study of Indian schoolchildren found that those who consumed less protein-rich foods like milk and legumes had higher levels of anxiety.[48] But since a true protein deficit isn't a huge concern for those who live in the developed world, it's more important to focus on the sources of protein and the amino acids that are their building blocks.

Plant versus Animal Protein

Another of the most contentious macronutrient debates is whether you should eat animal products or follow a strictly plant-based diet. The idea of eating a plant-based diet stretches back to ancient times. Greek philosophers like Pythagoras and Plato encouraged vegetarianism for moral and health reasons. Religions like Hinduism and Buddhism rejected the eating of animals. Thinkers from the Renaissance and the Enlightenment, including da Vinci, Rousseau, and Voltaire, also turned to vegetarianism. Centuries later, Albert Einstein would say that "nothing will increase the chances of survival for life on earth as much as the evolution to a vegetarian diet."[49] And since Einstein's time, we have come to understand far more fully how the mass-farming of livestock can promote animal cruelty and threaten the environment through unsustainable practices. Vegan diets, which totally eschew animal products, are a newer trend that has exploded in recent years. Veganism increased an estimated 600 percent from 2014 to 2018,[50] and the number of food and drink products that were labeled "plant-based" increased 287 percent from 2012 to 2018.[51] Based on what I see in my clinic — particularly among younger patients — I believe the movement toward plant-based diets will continue to grow.

Though I personally am a vegetarian, I respect everyone's individual food choices and acknowledge that meat and seafood bring their own nutritional strengths for those who choose to eat them. I simply don't see the wisdom in leaning into divisiveness. As a chef and a clinician, I choose to respect all foods, trying to account for environmental and social issues the best I can.

Recently, I have been aware of a steady march of recent headlines proclaiming that either meat eaters or vegetarians benefit from stronger mental health. These articles aren't always total bunk; they are often based on medical studies. For example, one meta-analysis found that meat eaters had lower anxiety and depression than vegans.[52] Another review claimed that vegans suffer from *less* stress and anxiety than omnivores.[53] And studies in France[54] and Australia[55] found no associations between vegetarian diets and altered anxiety levels.

As that broad range of study outcomes suggests, there is no definitive evidence for either a vegetarian or an omnivorous diet with respect to anxiety. That aligns with what I've seen in my more than twenty years of clinical experience. It's clear to me that for some, the psychological burden of eating animals — whether that concern stems from compassionate or environmental reasons — is simply too heavy to outweigh any possible benefit that could be gained from eating meat. I would never suggest that a committed vegetarian compromise their principles, because there are so many good ways to ensure that you are getting appropriate nutrition on a vegetarian diet.

If you choose to follow a vegetarian diet, it's important to account for any nutritional gaps your diet may have. For instance, we've already discussed that it can be difficult to get sufficient omega-3s without eating any fish, though a combination of plant-based foods rich in ALA like flaxseeds, walnuts, and soybeans, as well as a vegetarian algal supplement, can do the trick. In chapter 8, we will also see some ways in which eating a plant-based diet can risk shortages of some micronutrients.

If you choose to include animal protein in your diet, it's important to focus on moderate amounts of full-fat dairy, omega-3-rich fish, and high-quality sources of poultry, pork, and beef rather than greasy cheeseburgers and deep-fried chicken tenders. And meat should be accompanied by a range of whole grains, beans, lentils, colorful vegetables, and other plant-based foods that provide dietary fiber and anxiety-fighting compounds.

Amino Acids: Tryptophan and Glutamate

Just as fatty acids are the building blocks of fat, amino acids are the building blocks of protein. Your body takes in proteins through your food and breaks them down into amino acids that perform a huge number of tasks to keep your body running, including aiding in digestion, metabolism, growth, immunity, and mental health.

Tryptophan is an essential amino acid, meaning it's not produced naturally inside our bodies; it's available only through food. Tryptophan plays a variety of roles in our internal processes of protein synthesis and metabolism, but the most important for our purposes is that it is the precursor of serotonin. As we discussed in chapter 2, serotonin production relies on both a steady supply of dietary tryptophan and a healthy gut microbiome, and gut dysbiosis can affect how efficiently your body turns tryptophan into serotonin.[56]

While research into either restricting or supplementing tryptophan has proved its role in maintaining healthy serotonin levels, results have not always been straightforward when it comes to tryptophan's direct effect on anxiety. There have been studies that show reduced anxiety in a high-tryptophan diet compared to a low-tryptophan diet.[57] Older studies have found that taking a tryptophan supplement helps reduce anxiety but increasing dietary tryptophan does not,[58] while more recent studies have challenged this idea.[59] Yet another recent review found no correlation between low levels of tryptophan and anxiety.[60]

Despite the muddled evidence, I see enough of a clinical connection between anxiety, tryptophan, and the gut microbiome that I always recommend including tryptophan-rich proteins in your diet. Tryptophan is most abundant in poultry (I'm sure you have heard about the nap-inducing properties of Thanksgiving turkey), but it is also present in fish like tuna and salmon. Tryptophan can be found in plant sources, too, like soybeans and tofu, chickpeas, and pumpkin seeds.

In contrast to tryptophan, glutamic acid is a nonessential amino acid, meaning your body can synthesize it. Still, it is found in natural dietary sources like tomatoes and cheese, and in man-made seasonings in the form of monosodium glutamate, or MSG. You're probably familiar with MSG as an additive used to impart the umami flavor, enhancing the savory taste of dishes in a variety of Asian cuisines, as well as in condiments and snacks across the world. MSG developed a bad rap in the twentieth century, associated with a spurious condition called "Chinese restaurant syndrome," which supposedly caused headaches and other minor maladies; this never had much if any scientific grounding.[61]

Though MSG is now recognized as generally safe to eat, there is some possibility that it could increase anxiety. Like serotonin and GABA, glutamate is a neurotransmitter that's active in your brain. But serotonin and GABA are inhibitory neurotransmitters, calming your neurons from getting too worked up. Glutamate is an excitatory neurotransmitter, riling your neurons into action, so there is reason to believe that a surplus of it could keep your brain from calming down. Ongoing research is exploring the possibility of pharmaceuticals that alter glutamate transmission as a way of fighting anxiety, providing an alternative to SSRIs.[62] Moreover, there have been animal studies that link dietary glutamate to increased anxiety.[63]

However, other researchers have theorized that MSG's possible ill effects are more connected to the fact that it's often consumed as part of a diet full of processed foods.[64]

While I am following the research, I have not seen enough evidence to suggest totally avoiding glutamates. Still, in my clinic I discourage my patients from eating snack foods and takeout that are loaded with MSG; these foods are usually unhealthy choices that can worsen anxiety on their own. I also caution them about natural glutamates in tomatoes and mushrooms—despite being otherwise healthy whole foods, I've treated some individuals whose anxiety amps up after eating them. That's rare—these foods are the last ones to be eliminated if we are trialing foods to limit—but it's worth considering.

THE POWER OF MACRONUTRIENTS

We'll dive into specific eating plans and recipes in part 3, but you can already see the outlines of how the biggest components of your diet should come together. Though we are talking about the macronutrients as if they are totally separate, most foods contain more than one of them, and full meals should contain all three. You should always look for foods that cover as many healthy macronutrients as possible. For example, salmon is a great source of protein and of crucial omega-3 fats. Beans, lentils, and chickpeas are sources of both protein and carbohydrates that have healthy doses of dietary fiber. Avocado sourdough toast with a fried egg provides healthy MUFAs, medium-GI carbs rich in dietary fiber, and protein. Once you understand how the basics fit together, it's a fun—and delicious— puzzle to put together a fresh, wholesome, antianxiety diet.

Just as those foods consist of a combination of macronutrients, they're also full of other types of substances that are hugely important to your body—vitamins and minerals. Since these essential nutrients occur in much smaller quantities, we call them micronutrients, and they're our next area of focus.

CHAPTER EIGHT

Micronutrients

Indra was a twenty-five-year-old journalist who came to me to treat a persistent case of anxiety and exhaustion. Like many of us during the COVID-19 pandemic, Indra had gotten in the habit of staying indoors, spending most of her time on a laptop doing research and writing articles in her apartment. She kept active by following a home exercise plan on an app, so she wasn't entirely sedentary, but even after she was vaccinated and the worst of the pandemic had passed, she was finding herself anxious about the possibility of exercising outdoors. Furthermore, she had started to become increasingly fatigued to the point that it was interfering with her ability to meet deadlines. The specter of missed deadlines sparked more anxiety, as did the possibility that her freelance connections would dry up. It had all left Indra feeling like a shell of herself. At first, she attributed her symptoms to professional burnout, but as they worsened, she came to see me to evaluate possible dietary concerns.

As I took a detailed dietary history, I noticed that, unlike many of my patients, Indra did not have any obviously unhealthy components in her diet. In fact, she was extremely conscious about what she ate, having shifted to a fully plant-based diet while restaurants were closed during the pandemic. The balance and quantity of the macronutrients she was consuming were aligned with what I would suggest to a woman with her age and lifestyle. That made me realize that solving the problem might mean thinking *smaller*.

Several of Indra's symptoms raised concerns about deficiencies in vitamins and minerals. A combination of staying largely indoors, the cloudy Boston-area climate, and Indra's skin tone meant that a vitamin D deficiency could be a factor. A plant-based diet can also make it difficult to ensure proper levels of iron and vitamin B_{12}. I also wondered if her lack of vitality could be connected to low vitamin C — which can exacerbate low iron, since vitamin C helps with iron absorption.

We did a round of testing to check these parameters, and they all came back showing my hunches were correct: Indra was low on vitamins B_{12}, C, and D and was suffering from a case of iron-deficiency anemia. For iron and B_{12}, we turned to supplements to ensure she could get proper levels of them without consuming animal products, but I also recommended that she prioritize eating spinach and other leafy greens, up to 5 servings daily. She started to make a large mixed green salad every day and added vitamin C–packed red peppers, zests of lemon rind, and a squeeze of fresh lemon juice as her dressing. She ate kiwi a few times a week as dessert, another great source of vitamin C. For vitamin D, I encouraged her to spend at least ten minutes daily in the sun as the weather warmed, and I helped her incorporate sun-exposed mushrooms into her diet — keeping an eye on whether the glutamates in mushrooms worsened her anxiety, which they did not — and identify plant milks fortified with vitamin D without large amounts of added sugar.

Within a few weeks, Indra's anxiety eased and she started to feel energetic again. It took a few months to get her vitamin D levels up, but everything else normalized quickly. As her worry subsided and her vitality returned, she felt comfortable getting outdoors more often, practicing meditation again, and reactivating her gym membership, all of which helped her regain a fire for her work life.

It's incredible that substances found in such tiny amounts can have such a huge impact on health, but micronutrients are essential for proper functioning of enzymes, hormones, immunity, metabolism, and a wide variety of other biological processes throughout the body.[1] Furthermore, they play important roles in the brain, particularly in ensuring proper synthesis and release of neurotransmitters. Given what we know about how tightly intertwined these systems are, it becomes clearer why micronutrient deficits are a flashpoint for anxiety.

HOW MUCH DO I NEED?

As we explore micronutrients, we'll emphasize getting *enough* of various vitamins and minerals. But what *is* enough? That answer is quite variable, depending on the micronutrient in question as well as your gender, life stage, and other special circumstances. Men and women often have different micronutrient needs, as do younger and older people. Special subsets such as pregnant or lactating mothers often have their own unique requirements.

As you probably know, various health organizations publish guidelines to cover all these different cases. In this book, we'll use the dietary reference intakes, published by the Food and Nutrition Board of the National Academies of Science, Engineering, and Medicine. The key measure is the recommended dietary allowance (RDA) of different micronutrients, which provides a baseline for how much of each micronutrient the average person in each gender and age group needs to consume for optimal health. Complete information about RDAs can be found online at the National Institutes of Health Office of Dietary Supplements web page (https://ods .od.nih.gov/factsheets/list-all/).

While RDAs are valuable, in my clinical experience, I've learned that they are only a starting point. I always remind my patients that when adjusting micronutrient intake to fight anxiety, it's better to test levels and monitor anxiety symptoms as dietary changes are made, rather than exclusively adhering to RDAs.

NUTRIENT ABSORPTION

Another wrinkle in getting proper levels of micronutrients is that it's not just about how much you eat; it's about how much you absorb. Eating large amounts of vitamins and minerals doesn't really matter if your body is simply passing them through with other waste. Often, absorption decreases as you eat more of a given micronutrient—your body's natural way of regulating vitamin and mineral levels once your needs are met. But there may be other obstacles, including so-called antinutrients, specific compounds that hamper micronutrient absorption. For example, whole grains are a great source of many vitamins and minerals, but they also contain substances called phytates (or phytic acid), which can bind to minerals like calcium, iron, magnesium, and zinc in your gut. If the nutrients are bound by phytates, your gut can't absorb them. Phytates are also found in amaranth, legumes, nuts, and seeds. Similar effects occur with tannins in tea, coffee, and legumes, lectins and saponins in legumes and grains, oxalates in spinach and Swiss chard, and glucosinolates in vegetables like broccoli and Brussels sprouts.[2]

Types of Antinutrients

Antinutrient	Food Sources	Interferes with
Glucosinolates	Cruciferous vegetables: broccoli, Brussels sprouts, cabbage, cauliflower, kale	Absorption of iodine
Lectins	Legumes (beans, chickpeas, lentils), whole grains	Absorption of calcium, iron, and zinc
Oxalates	Leafy greens (especially spinach and Swiss chard), tea, beans, nuts, beets	Absorption of calcium

Phytates	Whole grains, seeds, legumes, nuts	Absorption of iron, zinc, magnesium, and calcium
Saponins	Whole grains, legumes	Absorption of vitamins A and E
Tannins	Tea, coffee, legumes	Absorption of iron

It's worth noting that antinutrients aren't harmful substances outside of potentially hampering mineral absorption, and you certainly shouldn't avoid foods that contain them, since cruciferous vegetables, whole grains, and legumes are some of the most powerful antianxiety foods you can eat. Even these antinutrient compounds are helpful to your body in various ways. For instance, phytates have been shown to be beneficial for lowering cholesterol and regulating blood sugar,[3] and in chapter 9 we'll learn about the antianxiety properties of the glucosinolates in cruciferous vegetables.

Antinutrients are a concern only if you're having trouble with a deficiency of specific vitamins and minerals. If that is the case, the problem can usually be worked around by planning out your meals and eating food in different combinations, for instance, avoiding phytate-rich grains in meals otherwise rich in minerals. Many food preparations, such as soaking, sprouting, or boiling, can also reduce antinutrient content.[4]

FORTIFIED AND ENRICHED FOODS

In the mid-twentieth century, when processed and packaged foods were rising to prominence, food scientists began to understand that processing techniques often rob food of its micronutrient value. For example, processing whole wheat into white flour reduces not only fiber but B vitamins and iron. To combat this, many producers add these micronutrients back in after processing to create "enriched" flour, enhancing the nutritional content. The Food and Drug Administration oversees this process and delineates guidelines for how much of each micronutrient should be added back into processed foods.

Historically, there has been evidence that fortification has helped deter certain conditions that stem from micronutrient deficiency.[5] But adding back nutrients doesn't make processed foods healthy. Given the wide variety of unprocessed food available today, I discourage getting micronutrients through fortified foods, particularly grains, for several reasons. While some nutrients are added back through the enrichment process, not all of them are—for instance, processors might add B vitamins and iron back to flour, but they are not adding fiber, zinc, or magnesium, all of which are also valuable. Perhaps even more important, the kinds of processed foods that are likely to be fortified do not lead to healthy eating patterns, and we have already learned that bad fats and added sugars can increase anxiety. As crucial as vitamins are, adding them to sugary breakfast cereal or packaged snacks does not make those foods less likely to worsen your risk of anxiety.

There are times when fortified foods can be useful, such as the fortified nut milks that Indra used to help increase her vitamin D levels. But in most cases, focusing on whole, unprocessed foods will ensure you are getting full, natural nutrition out of what you eat and will steer you away from eating unhealthy foods.

VITAMINS

The major goal of my work with Indra was to restore her *vitality*. It's no coincidence that "vitality" and "vitamin" share the same root word—the Latin "vita," which means life. Vitamins are organic compounds that are required for life. They are essential nutrients, meaning they can't be made by your body and therefore must come from dietary sources.

Humans require thirteen vitamins: four fat-soluble vitamins, A, D, E, K; and nine water-soluble vitamins, vitamin C and the eight B vitamins—thiamin (B_1), riboflavin (B_2), niacin (B_3), pantothenic acid (B$_5$), pyridoxine (B$_6$), biotin (B$_7$), folate (B$_9$), and cobalamin (B$_{12}$).

Fat-soluble vitamins are absorbed along with fats you eat, and excess amounts can be stored inside your liver and fatty tissues for months, keeping them available for later use. Excess water-soluble vitamins are flushed out of your system as you drink and urinate; they cannot be stored, meaning you require a daily supply to remain healthy.

The entire range of vitamins can influence anxiety, but I will focus on the most important for brain health: vitamins B, C, D, and E.

B Vitamins

The B vitamins can feel a little tricky to grasp since there are so many of them, each with both a name and a number. They were discovered and named during a flurry of vitamin research in the early twentieth century, and they were numbered in the order that they were officially recognized. The gaps in the numbering are a quirk of the definition of the word "vitamin" itself. There is a compound, adenine, that was discovered between B$_3$ and B$_5$. It would have become vitamin B$_4$, but further research determined that adenine can be synthesized within the body. Therefore, it doesn't count as a vitamin, and its number is skipped. The same is true of the compounds that would make up vitamins B$_8$, B$_{10}$, and B$_{11}$.

B vitamins play a significant role in maintaining healthy brain function, helping to provide energy and synthesize chemicals like the key neurotransmitters dopamine and serotonin, which can cause anxiety when disrupted.[6] B vitamins have also been shown to keep your brain young deeper into your life, improving cognition and discouraging degenerative brain conditions like dementia.[7]

The body of research on the role of different B vitamins in anxiety is not huge, but there are signs that nearly all of them are important. One cross-sectional population-based study showed that a moderate to high intake of B_1, B_3, B_5, and B_7 leads to lower levels of anxiety.[8] Another randomized controlled study found that high doses of B_6 and B_{12} showed some promise for reducing anxiety and depression.[9] Yet another study found that adults over sixty who were in the lowest 20 percent of levels of B_2, B_6, and B_9 were more likely to be depressed, and those deficient in B_6 had increased anxiety.[10]

While some studies and reviews have not been quite as definitive,[11] I believe that B vitamins should be on the radar of anyone suffering from anxiety, especially since most of them are plentiful in otherwise nutritious food that shouldn't be difficult to add to your diet.

Foods that contain B vitamins: The B vitamins often appear together in many foods, like whole grains, leafy greens, nuts, seeds, meat, poultry, and fish.[12]

- Vitamin B_1 (thiamin) is found in lean pork and beef (especially liver), wheat germ and whole grains, eggs, fish, legumes, and nuts. Thiamin is very sensitive to food preparation, including grain processing, soaking, and even high-heat cooking. Because of this, thiamin is often added back into processed foods, but it's always better to get it from unprocessed, whole sources.

- Vitamin B_2 (riboflavin) is found in dairy (though reduced-fat dairy has lower riboflavin content), fatty fish, and certain fruits and vegetables, especially dark green vegetables. Many processed grains are also fortified with B_2, but I prefer to focus on unprocessed sources.

- Vitamin B_3 (niacin) is found in beef, pork, poultry, fish, nuts, legumes, and grains. Forms of niacin found in animal products (and those used to fortify processed grains) are easier for your body to process, so it may be a bit harder to ensure proper niacin levels in those on a plant-based diet. You may also want to discuss a supplement with your doctor.

- Vitamin B_5 (pantothenic acid) is found in beef, poultry, mushrooms, avocados, nuts, seeds, milk, yogurt, potatoes, eggs, brown rice, oats, and broccoli.

- Vitamin B_6 (pyridoxine) is found in meat, fish, nuts, beans, grains, fruits, and vegetables. It is also heavily featured in many multivitamins and added as a supplement to a variety of processed foods.

- Vitamin B_7 (biotin) is found in beef liver, pork, eggs, salmon, avocados, sweet potatoes, and nuts. Biotin is often marketed as a supplement to treat hair loss and promote healthy skin and nails.

- Vitamin B_9 (folate) is found in liver, seafood, eggs, whole grains, dark leafy vegetables, fresh fruit, beans, peanuts, and sunflower seeds. Folate is particularly important to pregnant women to reduce the risk of certain birth defects, so in 1998, the Food and Drug Administration began requiring manufacturers to fortify enriched grains with it. Most people should be able to get enough folate through normal dietary sources, but it's recommended that pregnant women also take a folic acid supplement.

- Vitamin B_{12} (cobalamin) is found in animal products like meat, eggs, and dairy. Because of this, it can be a challenge for those on plant-based diets. B_{12} can also be difficult to absorb; it relies on a protein called an intrinsic factor to be properly processed in the gut. The B_{12} in supplements is formulated in a way to make it easier to absorb, so it may make sense to consider that route.

Vitamin C

Vitamin C might be the best-known vitamin, due to the popular idea (first championed by famous chemist Linus Pauling) that large doses of it help prevent the common cold and other seasonal diseases. While this association isn't totally backed up by science — a prominent review showed that colds were no less likely in study participants who took extra vitamin C, though symptoms weren't quite as severe and didn't last quite as long[13] — there's no doubt that vitamin C contributes to overall immune function and assists with a variety of metabolic processes. A severe deficit of vitamin C famously leads to the hemorrhagic disease scurvy, which causes bleeding gums and poor wound healing.

Vitamin C is active in the brain, particularly as an antioxidant, protecting the brain against oxidative stress caused by dangerous free radicals.[14] Like the B vitamins, vitamin C also plays a significant role in neurotransmitter synthesis and regulation, particularly concerning dopamine.[15]

Studies have shown that vitamin C promotes mental vitality, reducing fatigue and improving mood.[16] Other studies have explored how the antioxidant properties of vitamin C can help ease the burden of stress-related diseases like anxiety and depression.[17] A double-blind randomized controlled trial also found that vitamin C supplementation directly reduced anxiety levels.[18]

Foods that contain vitamin C: Citrus fruits are a great source of vitamin C, but surprisingly, higher amounts are found in kiwi and red bell peppers. It's also found in berries, tomatoes, potatoes, and green leafy vegetables. Vitamin C can be destroyed by high heat and leached off into cooking liquids during boiling or simmering. Therefore, it's better to use quicker cooking methods like stir-frying and blanching, or, better yet, to eat ripe vitamin C–rich fruits and vegetables raw.[19]

Vitamin D

Vitamin D is best known as the "sunshine vitamin," and indeed, it's the only vitamin that our bodies can synthesize on their own, through a reaction in our skin when exposed to UV rays from the sun. However, as we saw with Indra, skin color, climate, latitude, sunscreen usage, and an indoor-focused lifestyle can all be obstacles to healthy levels of vitamin D. As a result, an estimated 77 percent of Americans are vitamin D deficient.[20] That means everyone should be trying to get as much vitamin D as possible from every source, especially through the food you eat. Since the best sources of vitamin D are fish, meat, and dairy, those who are on a plant-based diet will want to consider a supplement, which you should discuss with your doctor.

Vitamin D performs many important functions throughout your body, helping to build strong bones by allowing the body to absorb calcium (which we'll talk about later in the chapter), reducing inflammation, and boosting immune function. In the brain, vitamin D has been shown to be neuroprotective, protecting against cognitive decline.[21] As with other vitamins, vitamin D is involved with neurotransmitter production and regulation and has an effect on glutamine, norepinephrine, dopamine, and serotonin.[22]

Vitamin D has been shown to reduce negative emotions brought on by depression and anxiety,[23] and lower levels of vitamin D have been shown to correlate with both conditions.[24] Increasing vitamin D levels in patients who are deficient has been shown to reduce anxiety.[25] In another study, GAD patients who were given vitamin D supplements showed improved symptoms compared to controls.[26]

Vitamin D is most effective at fighting anxiety in those who are already extremely deficient in vitamin D,[27] but given how common vitamin D deficiency is in our society, I feel strongly that anyone suffering from anxiety should make a conscious effort to eat as much vitamin D as possible, or consider the possibility of a supplement.[28]

Foods that contain vitamin D: Your body's ability to make its own vitamin D from sun exposure complicates pinpointing exactly how much of it you need to take in through dietary sources. But given its importance, I think everyone should get as much as possible from food. The best food sources of vitamin D are fatty fish, liver, eggs, and certain sun-exposed mushrooms. Many foods are also fortified with vitamin D, including grains and dairy. Cod liver oil is a great source of vitamin D. Vitamin D is also available in other supplements, which are worth discussing with your doctor if you feel like you're at risk of vitamin D deficiency due to lack of sun exposure.

Vitamin E

Vitamin E is particularly important to your immune function. Like vitamin C, vitamin E is a powerful antioxidant that binds to harmful free radicals, protecting your cells from oxidative stress. These antioxidant properties are particularly important in the brain, where oxidative stress is especially dangerous, increasing in severity as we age. Sure enough, high levels of vitamin E have been firmly associated with better cognitive performance in older people, and it has been studied as a possible treatment for Alzheimer's disease.[29]

Animal studies have also suggested that vitamin E deficiency can lead to anxiety.[30] Though one review of human studies came up a bit mixed,[31] vitamin E has been shown to alleviate chronic inflammation and improve metabolic disorders like metabolic syndrome, both of which we know are connected to anxiety.[32]

Foods that contain vitamin E: The richest sources of vitamin E are vegetable oils like sunflower, safflower, soybean, palm, and peanut oil. Unfortunately, as we covered in chapter 7, these omega-6 PUFA–rich oils aren't healthy to consume in large quantities, so it's important to look to other sources. Vitamin E can also be found in almonds, peanuts, hazelnuts, and leafy greens.

MINERALS

I once had a friend whose new puppy was adorable in every way, except that he was entirely too keen on eating rocks, constantly on the hunt for gravel to put in his mouth. My friend was diligent about not letting the pup swallow them, and a bit exasperated that she was constantly on her knees, prying another pebble out of her beloved pet's mouth. I tried to console her that even though he was going about it the wrong way, he had the right idea: we *all* eat rocks, if in extremely tiny quantities. And these essential dietary minerals are crucial to good health.

The National Institutes of Health identifies fifteen minerals that are key to health, but we will focus on the five that are most tightly tied to anxiety: calcium, iron, magnesium, manganese, and zinc. We'll review them in alphabetical order.

Calcium

Calcium is the most abundant mineral in the body. It makes up a large proportion of your bones and teeth, providing their rigidity. There is also a small amount of calcium in your blood and tissues, which helps with the functioning of your blood vessels, muscles, nerves, and hormones. Calcium is involved in several aspects of brain function, including the synthesis and release of neurotransmitters like serotonin.

A 2022 study of 1,233 American college students[33] and a 2020 study of college students in Jordan[34] found that higher calcium intake was correlated with lower stress, positive mood, and reduced anxiety. Low calcium intake has also been associated with poor sleep quality, which has been found to correlate with anxiety.[35]

Foods that contain calcium: The best sources of calcium are dairy products like milk, yogurt, and cheese. Of course, many people are lactose intolerant and cannot consume dairy, or they avoid it because they follow a plant-based diet. Luckily, there are plenty of other sources of calcium, including nuts, seeds, peas, beans, and fish. Consider that in the United States and Western Europe, well over half of most people's calcium intake is from dairy, but in China, only around 7 percent comes from dairy, with most of it coming from vegetables and legumes.

Iron

Iron is one of the best-known dietary minerals for good reason: iron deficiency is the most common nutritional deficiency in the world. The resulting condition, iron deficiency anemia, is a serious health threat, particularly to women and children.

The classic role of iron in your body is in your blood, where iron-rich hemoglobin allows your red blood cells to carry oxygen throughout your tissue. But iron also plays an important role in the brain. Iron deficiency in pregnant mothers can lead to a premature birth and low birth weight, both of which can result in long-term complications. Iron is also a key to healthy neurotransmitter metabolism, with iron levels playing a role in the availability of neurotransmitters like serotonin and dopamine, as well as affecting levels of GABA.[36]

Human and animal studies have linked iron deficiency with anxiety, among other psychiatric disorders, particularly in infants, children, and adolescents.[37] Iron deficiency early in life can continue to cause trouble in the brain for many years, long after iron levels return to a healthy level, so it's particularly important to make sure that infants and children get the recommended amount of iron.[38]

It's worth noting that some animal studies have shown that a *surplus* of iron in the brain can cause anxiety symptoms.[39] While this is a consideration when taking iron supplements (working with a doctor to monitor this is key), it's hard to consume that much iron from dietary sources — another example of why it's preferable to get nutrients from food sources rather than supplements.

Foods that contain iron: Meat is the best source of iron, since it has high levels in the form of hemoglobin, which is easy for our bodies to absorb. Liver is the most iron-rich cut of meat, but if you don't have a taste for organ meat, beef has the highest iron content, followed by pork. Chicken and fish also contain iron, though at slightly lower levels.

As we saw with Indra, iron can be a bit trickier to get on a plant-based diet. Plants offer many sources of iron, including leafy greens like spinach and chard, whole grains, nuts, and berries. Unfortunately, the iron in plant-based foods is harder for our bodies to absorb, so even if you're eating generous amounts of plant-based sources of iron, you may still have an iron deficiency. Complicating matters further, antinutrients and other chemicals in dairy and soy products can inhibit iron absorption. Luckily, there are some nutrients, like vitamin C, that do promote iron absorption.

Given the difficulties of getting enough iron in a plant-based diet, I often recommend that my vegetarian patients (particularly women of childbearing age) take an iron supplement, as I did with Indra. Since iron supplements can cause some side effects — especially upset stomach — it's best to consult with your doctor to determine the proper dosage.

Magnesium

Magnesium is active throughout your body, facilitating more than three types of enzymatic action that help you build strong bones, create energy, and regulate blood sugar and blood pressure. Its role in metabolism explains why magnesium deficiency is often associated with conditions like type 2 diabetes.[40] Magnesium can be a bit tough to measure, since most of it is tied up in your bones and cells rather than floating freely in the blood where it can be easily tested. Still, researchers estimate that magnesium deficiency is quite widespread, with up to 60 percent of Americans not consuming enough.[41]

In the brain, magnesium assists with myelination (the formation and maintenance of the junctions between nerve cells called synapses) and with regulation of neurotransmitters like glutamate and serotonin.[42] Research on magnesium's role in mood disorders was originally focused on depression, and a variety of studies have shown that low magnesium levels can lead to depression and that supplementation can improve symptoms.[43] There is also evidence that magnesium levels affect the stress response and that stress can actually deplete magnesium in your body.[44] A systematic review of the effects of magnesium on anxiety found that about half the relevant studies showed that magnesium improved anxiety symptoms.[45] Even though results are somewhat mixed, given magnesium's significance in so many anxiety-adjacent conditions, I strongly recommend ensuring that you eat enough magnesium-rich foods.

Foods that contain magnesium: Magnesium is found primarily in whole grains, legumes, nuts, and dark chocolate. Vegetables, fruit, meats, and fish also have magnesium, though at lower levels.

The importance of eating whole grains for their anxiety benefit is particularly crucial with regard to magnesium. Refining and processing grains drastically reduces magnesium levels, with white flour and rice having approximately 80 percent less magnesium than whole wheat flour and brown rice.[46]

Manganese

Manganese also plays a role in many of the body's enzymatic actions, assisting with bone formation, metabolism, and antioxidant processes. Magnesium and manganese have more in common than just their names — their properties are so similar that many enzymes can function using either one, though there are roles that are unique to manganese.[47]

Unlike magnesium, manganese deficiency is extremely rare, and in fact, the greater concern is *over*exposure. An overabundance of manganese in the brain has been associated with neurological disorders similar to Parkinson's disease[48] as well as increased anxiety in both animal and human studies.[49] Despite this association, manganese overexposure tends to be associated with environmental factors, like working in manganese-rich environments, and it's doubtful that you would get too much manganese from a normal diet. Still, that's another illustration of the potential danger of getting too much of certain micronutrients from supplements.

Foods that contain manganese: Manganese is primarily found in whole grains, rice, and nuts. Dark chocolate, tea, mussels, clams, legumes, fruit, leafy vegetables (spinach), seeds (flax, sesame, pumpkin, sunflower, and pine nuts), and spices (chili powder, cloves, and saffron) are also rich in manganese.

Zinc

Zinc is another mineral that is active throughout the body, assisting with enzymatic activity and enhancing the immune system—you may recognize zinc as an additive in some over-the-counter cold remedies.

Zinc is prominent in your brain, performing several roles to promote optimal brain function, including spurring the growth of new neurons—particularly in anxiety hot spots like the hippocampus—and mediating inflammation and oxidation.[50] Zinc is also crucial to the pituitary gland, a central component of the HPA-axis that helps control mood regulation, and zinc deficiency can result in a range of abnormal behaviors.[51]

Zinc has been found to be effective in treating certain types of depression and has also been shown to enhance the effects of antidepressant drugs in treatment-resistant patients.[52] Studies have also shown that anxiety sufferers have lower levels of zinc than controls.[53] Zinc deficiency was also correlated with both depression and anxiety in a study of female high school students[54] and a study of adults age sixty and over,[55] indicating that it is important in all stages of brain development.

Foods that contain zinc: The richest food sources of zinc are meat, fish, and seafood — oysters contain more zinc per serving than any other food. If fresh oysters are unavailable, canned oysters are an option. Eggs and dairy also contain zinc. Beans, nuts, and whole grains contain zinc, too, but it's not as easy to absorb from plant sources due to their phytate content, as we discussed earlier in the chapter.

SMART SUPPLEMENTATION

When it comes to getting the correct level of micronutrients, I am always a proponent of food first. As long as you are eating a healthy diet full of whole foods, there is a good chance you won't need to take a regimen of supplements. However, there are certainly times when dietary restrictions, interactions with other drugs, or differences in physiology can mean that diet alone doesn't ensure sufficient levels of certain micronutrients. When such gaps occur in our nutrition, supplements can be an important part of lowering anxiety.

My golden rule for supplementation is "test, don't guess." Before beginning to take any supplement, have your doctor test your micronutrient levels. If you are low in any vitamins or minerals, first try to make up the deficit with food. If you don't see the desired results on follow-up tests, consider a supplement. The most common micronutrient deficiencies I see in my clinic are found in the following table. Remember that RDAs can vary by gender, age, and a variety of other factors. The specifics can be found at the National Institutes of Health Office of Dietary Supplements web page (https://ods.od.nih.gov/factsheets/list-all/).

Micronutrient	Who Should Test?	Tips
B complex vitamins	Those who follow a plant-based diet are at risk of low B complex levels, especially B_{12}, since most food sources are of animal origin.	Supplements are available that cover the entire B complex. With your doctor's help, decide whether to take a full B complex supplement or a specific B vitamin. Since B vitamins are water-soluble, the body excretes excess amounts in urine, so there is relatively low risk of overdoing it. However, excessively high doses of B vitamins can still be dangerous and can interact with certain medications, so talk to your doctor about risk factors.
Vitamin D	The chief risk factor for vitamin D deficiency is lack of sun exposure, particularly for those with darker skin tones. Vegetarians and vegans are also at risk, because dietary vitamin D sources are largely from seafood and fortified dairy.	Vitamin D is stored in body fat and can be toxic in excess. Given interactions with vitamin D, magnesium, and calcium, I often recommend supplementing them together.
Magnesium	Magnesium is difficult to test, since the bulk of it is tied up in your bones, with only roughly 1 percent circulating in your blood. Discuss the possibilities for testing with your health practitioner.	There are several types of magnesium supplements, but for mental health I generally recommend magnesium bisglycinate or magnesium L-threonate. Magnesium can interact with a range of prescription drugs, so talk to your doctor about risk factors.

Calcium	Calcium deficiency is most common in those who do not eat dairy. Women are more likely to suffer from calcium deficiency than men.	Calcium can interact with prescription medicines, including antibiotics and blood pressure medication, so talk to your doctor about risk factors.
Iron	Vegetarians and vegans are at heightened risk of iron deficiency because plant-based iron is more difficult for your body to absorb than the iron found in animal products.	Iron supplements are less easily tolerated than other supplements, so work with your doctor to find the correct formulation and dosage. Vitamin C can increase iron absorption from plant-based dietary sources, but studies show that it is not necessary to pair a vitamin C supplement with an iron supplement.[56]

BIG THINGS COME IN SMALL PACKAGES

I could write an entire book on micronutrients' role in mental health, so this is not an exhaustive review. For instance, there have been indications that vitamins A[57] and K[58] are also linked to anxiety, as are minerals like copper[59] and selenium.[60] But the key message is that even these tiny dietary components can have a massive effect on mental health and offer ways to calm your mind with food.

Vitamins and minerals aren't the only compounds that can make a big difference in fighting anxiety. In the next chapter, we'll learn about the world of bioactives, phytochemicals, and herbal supplements.

CHAPTER NINE

Bioactives and Herbal Medicine

Naomi was a twenty-three-year-old woman who was suffering from a host of symptoms: digestive issues, headaches, fatigue, and insomnia. She told me that she often felt like her body was falling apart. Her primary care physician had referred her to me after ruling out serious physical conditions, suspecting that anxiety might be at the root of her symptoms. Naomi was skeptical, since she hadn't been experiencing any strong anxious feelings, but I explained to her how somatic anxiety can be responsible for problems in the body, even in the absence of the classic mental symptoms. Gradually, she agreed that it was worth pursuing treatments for anxiety.

Naomi's diet was already in good order, with a healthy balance of macronutrients and micronutrients, so there weren't any major changes to be made there. She was totally opposed to trying any kind of pharmaceutical. Both SSRIs and benzodiazepines were out of the question, since she didn't want to use medication for a condition she wasn't sure she had. I realized we would have to get a bit creative.

When patients approach me with anxiety symptoms, I do not generally prescribe herbal supplements as first-line treatments, but given the limitations of Naomi's case, it felt reasonable to try. I suggested trying an oral supplement of lavender oil, a natural herbal preparation that has been shown to improve symptoms of somatic anxiety without causing serious side effects or drowsiness.[1]

Though lavender isn't commonly used in cooking beyond flavorings in teas and baked goods, it has been used as a scent in perfumes and soaps since the Middle Ages and is a popular component of alternative treatments like aromatherapy massages. While there is some anecdotal evidence that lavender can ease anxiety through its scent, the evidence isn't ironclad.[2] However, lavender oil is also available in an oral supplement—notably in a preparation called Silexan, a government-approved medication in Germany, and as an herbal remedy in the United States. Silexan has shown promising results in clinical trials as an antianxiety treatment,[3] likely due to the way it binds to serotonin receptors in the brain.[4]

Naomi did her own careful research, which helped her feel more in control, and settled on a clean supplement that contained only lavender oil. We agreed this was a safe option for her. After two weeks on an intermediate dose of lavender oil capsules, Naomi's symptoms began to improve, and before long they disappeared entirely. This isn't always the case—I've had patients who didn't see results from herbal medication until six to eight weeks, often with adjustments in dosage made along the way—but I was delighted that Naomi was able to find relief so quickly without using pharmaceuticals. While she also took up acupuncture again, along with tai chi—both of which helped her relax and feel more at ease—the initial results came after using the supplement, and these were the supporting act. Once she saw how effective the herbal treatment was, she became even more committed to an integrated and holistic approach to fend off her anxiety.

WHAT ARE BIOACTIVES?

Despite its roots in folk medicine, the effectiveness of lavender oil isn't due to mysticism or magic. Just like pharmaceuticals, it's effective because it contains chemicals that exert an impact on the biological mechanics of your brain or body. These chemicals are called bioactives, and they have gained prominence as an area of research and in the medical community in recent years. Bioactives are a broad, complex category of chemicals, so we will only be able to scratch the surface, but in this chapter, we will explore their potential to relieve anxiety, whether found in foods we eat or in herbal supplements.

Bioactives appear in only trace amounts in food and herbs, but they can have an outsize effect on health. If that reminds you of the micronutrients we discussed in chapter 8, that's no coincidence. There is no official consensus, but some experts classify vitamins and minerals as types of bioactives. Others make a key distinction: unlike micronutrients, bioactives are not specifically *required* by your body. While their presence may help you maintain optimal health, their absence isn't going to keep your body from functioning normally. For example, if you have a severe shortage of iron or vitamin C, your body will gradually succumb to conditions like anemia and scurvy. The lavender oil that helped Naomi wasn't essential to her health; it simply bolstered her brain and body against her somatic anxiety.

While vitamins and minerals come from a broad range of plant and animal sources, almost all bioactives are phytochemicals, meaning they are produced by plants ("phyto" is the Greek word for plant). The vast range of plants we can eat or turn into herbal preparations means there are a multitude of bioactives that have different biological effects, ranging from the antioxidants in berries to the caffeine in coffee and tea to the opioids in addictive drugs. Trying to learn the specifics of every bioactive compound, what their effects are, and what foods contain them can feel like a Sisyphean effort of confusing terminology (for example, a class of phytochemicals called flavonoids is further divided into flavones, flavonols, flavanones, flavanonols, and flavanols, among a few others[5] — not exactly designed to be distinctive and easy to remember).

Rather than getting too lost in the jargon, we will discuss the potential of bioactives to fight anxiety in two main groups: those that are concentrated in certain phytochemical-rich foods and those that may be worth incorporating into your routine via herbal supplements.

BIOACTIVES IN FOOD

Everyone knows you should eat your vegetables. In the previous two chapters, we've discussed how fruits and vegetables are packed with helpful macro- and micronutrients, but they are also a key source of dietary bioactives. This is another reason why it's so important that fresh fruits and vegetables make up a large proportion of your diet.

The most common type of bioactives found in fruits and vegetables is polyphenols, a group of phytochemicals known for their powerful antioxidant properties. Polyphenols have been found to have a range of positive effects on health, including decreased risk of heart disease and stroke, protection against neurodegenerative diseases, and improved metabolic indicators like blood pressure and lipids.[6] As we've seen in many cases throughout this book, foods that correct metabolic imbalances and decrease inflammatory disease also tend to reduce anxiety. Polyphenols have also been shown to help promote a healthy gut microbiome, which, as we know, is an essential part of calming your mind.[7]

Studies on polyphenol supplementation and anxiety have been somewhat mixed—a 2021 meta-analysis found polyphenols helpful in depression,[8] but with no strong improvement in anxiety, whereas a 2022 meta-analysis found benefits for both conditions.[9] But it's also important to consider a large body of research that has correlated eating lots of fruits and vegetables with better mental well-being and lower anxiety scores. For example, in the Lettuce Be Happy study, British researchers followed participants for seven years, tracking their diets and mental health, finding that those who ate the most fruits and vegetables tended to be the happiest, and even a modest increase in fruit and vegetable consumption had a large positive effect.[10] While such studies don't tie these improvements directly to polyphenols, I feel confident that they are a part of the picture, alongside vitamins, minerals, and dietary fiber.

Because there are so many varieties of polyphenols in fruits and vegetables, you shouldn't get too hung up on trying to trace which compound is found in which specific food. Instead, the best way to ensure that you're getting a range of polyphenols is to eat a widely varied diet that incorporates all kinds of different fruits and vegetables. One good rule of thumb is to eat fruits and vegetables of many different colors — those with rich colors are particularly rich in polyphenols. Think of the reds and blues of berries, the oranges and yellows of citrus fruits and carrots, the deep greens of kale and spinach, and the vibrant purple of eggplant.

Berries are particularly well known for their antioxidant properties, protecting the brain from oxidative stress.[11] Most of the research into the positive effects of berries has centered on their potential to protect against neurodegenerative diseases, such as Alzheimer's and Parkinson's, but given that neuroprotective foods often seem to improve anxiety, I'm confident in recommending them — especially since they have a low glycemic index and can deliver a sweet, satisfying treat without negatively affecting metabolic health when eaten in moderation, about ¼ cup to ½ cup a day.

A new favorite vegetable of mine is purple sprouting broccoli, a beautiful purple form of broccoli I was introduced to when I visited London. Thanks to the anthocyanins that give it its purple color, it has almost double the antioxidant polyphenol content of regular green broccoli, which is already an amazing source of nutrients.[12] (See the recipe for Pan-Seared Purple Sprouting Broccoli on page 260.)

Cruciferous vegetables like purple sprouting broccoli, along with green broccoli, Brussels sprouts, collard greens, kale, and other vegetables also contain bioactives called glucosinolates, which give them their bitter taste and odor.[13] Research has shown that glucosinolates are key in the prevention and treatment of several chronic diseases. Specifically, studies show that cruciferous vegetables can help improve blood sugar regulation and blood pressure, which can help fight against metabolic disorders. Glucosinolates can also improve psychiatric conditions such as depression, anxiety, autism, and Alzheimer's disease, as well as immune disorders such as multiple sclerosis, and a particular compound called sulforaphane has shown potential in fighting cancer.[14] I was first alerted to the incredible benefits of this food group when I battled breast cancer. Human studies have shown that exposure to sulforaphane helps slow breast cancer progression, arresting the cancer cell cycle and discouraging metastasis.[15]

While you may need to visit a farmers' market to find purple sprouting broccoli (or grow it yourself!), I have high hopes that this beautiful, delicious, and brain-healthy choice will become more commonly available as its positive effects are studied further. In the meantime, I encourage you to take advantage of the polyphenols, glucosinolates, and other bioactives in cruciferous vegetables like green broccoli, cauliflower, Brussels sprouts, and cabbage.

In addition to a wide variety of fruits and vegetables, there are several foods and beverages that are known to be bursting with polyphenols and other helpful bioactives, including tea, chocolate, wine, and various herbs and spices. Unlike fruits and vegetables, some of these foods and drinks are easy to overindulge in, so let's consider the pluses and minuses of each one.

Tea

Tea has been used to improve mood and soothe worry for thousands of years, and a steaming cup of tea certainly helps me to calm my mind. Modern medical research has backed up this association, as tea contains polyphenols that can help relieve anxiety. Of course, tea isn't monolithic, and different black, green, and herbal tea preparations have varying effects on mental health.

Black tea is the most prominent type of tea in the United States and Europe and is popular across the globe. The crucial polyphenols in black tea are theaflavins, which have been shown to have antioxidant and antibacterial properties. Theaflavins have also been shown to ease anxiety symptoms in animal studies, likely via spurring the release of dopamine.[16] Black tea has also been shown to assist with recovery from stress and boost relaxation.[17] Even just inhaling the aroma of black tea has been shown to ease feelings of stress and reduce stress markers found in saliva.[18]

Green tea is popular in Asia as both traditionally brewed tea and the ground powdered preparation called matcha. Green tea is increasingly prevalent throughout the world, as it has been recognized for its good health effects, including boosts to mood and cognition.[19] The most important bioactive in green tea is L-theanine, an amino acid that has been shown to reduce feelings of stress and anxiety.[20]

It's important to remember that both black and green tea contain caffeine, a familiar bioactive compound that is part of the alkaloid group. Caffeine has a somewhat complicated relationship with mental health. I think many of us can attest that caffeine in moderation is a net positive for our ability to function in a busy, fast-moving world. But it's important not to go overboard. High levels of caffeine consumption can lead to an increase in anxiety symptoms and even to serious events like panic attacks, especially in people already suffering from anxiety disorders like GAD and panic disorder.[21] My recommendation is to keep caffeine consumption under 400 mg/day. One cup of black tea contains about 47 mg of caffeine, and 1 cup of green tea contains about 28 mg,[22] so it's unlikely that you'd exceed the limit while drinking only tea. But be careful if you're also drinking coffee or other beverages that contain caffeine.

I also want to note that tea recommendations are focused on plain, steeped tea, not tea drinks with tons of added unhealthy fats and sugars or nonnutritive sweeteners. These additives can easily overpower the positive benefits of tea. A 2021 study found that regular drinkers of sugary bubble tea are more likely to suffer from depression and anxiety;[23] that study meshes with my clinical experience, as we saw with my bubble tea–loving patient Mary in chapter 3. (See the recipe for Matcha Green "Bubble" Tea on page 268 for an alternative.)

Herbal teas generally do not contain caffeine, and certain preparations have been shown to ease anxiety. For example, rosemary tea has shown promising antianxiety effects.[24] Given Naomi's success at battling her anxiety with lavender oil, it's no surprise that lavender tea has also been found to help.[25] The classic chamomile tea has been shown to significantly reduce symptoms of GAD.[26] And the South African herbal tea rooibos has been shown to have powerful antioxidant properties, especially when steeped for long periods to boost the polyphenol content.[27]

Chocolate

Chocolate is another food that's thought of as a mood enhancer, though often for more indulgent reasons than tea — rich, sweet, high-calorie chocolate candies are popular forms of comfort food that put taste and satisfaction over health concerns. But while most chocolate candy isn't good for you, that's more the fault of the sugar and unhealthy fats than of the chocolate itself. Dark chocolate that has less sugar and greater cacao concentration contains a wealth of polyphenols with the potential to improve anxiety.

A 2022 meta-analysis concluded that cacao-rich products spurred significant improvement in anxiety symptoms in the short term (studies were too sparse to make a conclusion about long-term effects).[28] Dark chocolate has been shown to reduce stress chemicals and help regulate the gut microbiome in anxious study participants.[29] Furthermore, chocolate has shown potential in increasing positive mood states[30] and protecting against depression.[31] Clinically I've seen the benefit in anxiety-ridden patients who were accustomed to sugary desserts that made their anxiety worse. Acquiring a taste for extra-dark chocolate as a replacement for sweeter options helped lower their symptoms.

I want to stress that these findings aren't an excuse to eat every candy bar you can get your hands on. The ill effects of eating too much sugar can certainly outweigh chocolate's positive effects, especially since sweeter milk chocolate has lower amounts of helpful polyphenols. Even some dark chocolate can be high in added sugars, so make sure you focus on high-quality, cacao-rich, minimally sweetened extra-dark chocolate.

Red Wine

Wine is rich in polyphenols and antioxidants that can have positive effects on health. Moderate consumption of red wine has long been associated with improved cognition and neuroprotection.[32] The polyphenol resveratrol can help regulate the release of neurotransmitters like serotonin and dopamine.

Again, moderation is key. Overconsumption of alcohol is a serious problem. Alcohol abuse has been found to be highly concurrent with anxiety disorders, and the two can worsen each other. No amount of polyphenols is going to overcome the damage that drinking too much can cause, so if you're going to drink, limit your consumption and pay close attention to how you feel after consuming alcohol. If you'd rather avoid drinking wine but don't want to miss out on the helpful effects of resveratrol, it's worth speaking to your doctor about a resveratrol supplement.

Herbs and Spices

Turmeric is known as a brain-healthy spice due to its high levels of curcumin, a bright yellow phenolic compound that is used in cooking and as an herbal remedy in Ayurvedic traditions. Curcumin is most often suggested as a possible treatment for depression, due to how it increases levels of brain chemicals like monoamines and brain-derived neurotrophic factor; it also reduces inflammation and helps reverse metabolic abnormalities.[33] However, recent studies have shown positive effects on anxiety too, with some finding that curcumin is even more effective at treating anxiety than at treating depression.[34] When cooking with turmeric, it's important to include black pepper, which has been shown to make it easier for your body to absorb curcumin, multiplying its effects.[35]

Saffron is another seasoning that garners a lot of attention as a possible anxiety reducer. Saffron contains around 150 phytochemicals that have antioxidant and anti-inflammatory properties, including several that have been shown to be helpful for reducing anxiety.[36] A meta-analysis of twenty-three studies on saffron's effect on depression and anxiety found that it had a large positive effect on both conditions.[37]

Other herbs like rosemary,[38] an Indian variety of basil called tulsi, or "holy basil,"[39] and oregano[40] have also been shown to help reduce stress and alleviate anxiety. But while cooking with these herbs and spices is never a bad idea, it's a challenge to get large enough amounts of them into your diet. Since bioactives occur only in tiny amounts, and we generally season our food with small amounts of herbs and spices, it's not practical to try to get enough of an herb or spice through your cooking to make a difference. I once had a patient who was delighted that I mentioned the positive effects of saffron, because she loved to cook pastas and rice dishes that were flavored with it. But once we broke down the amount of saffron she would need to eat to get the recommended dosage — it takes around twenty-one threads of saffron to yield the same effect as a 50 mg saffron supplement — she agreed that it would be more sensible (and more cost-effective, as saffron is very expensive) to look to a supplement. She ended up having a positive response to the supplement, lowering her anxiety within six weeks, and continued to cook with saffron on the side.

For this reason, while I certainly encourage you to cook with a broad range of herbs and spices in order to reap the benefits of their phytochemical content, if you want to try a regimen of a specific compound to target your anxiety, it's often best to work with a holistic medicine or integrative medicine practitioner to determine a quality supplement and an appropriate dose.

That is a good note on which to shift our discussion to the topic of herbal medicine.

BIOACTIVES IN HERBAL MEDICINE

Herbal medicine has deep roots all over the world, with herbs playing a major role in allopathic, Ayurvedic, and Eastern medicine. Many people don't know that as late as 1890, 59 percent of American pharmaceutical products were based on herbs or herbal combinations.[41] Even today, herbal medicine is the most common form of alternative medicine, with an estimated 20 percent of Americans taking herbal medications to treat or prevent diseases.[42] While some practitioners of conventional medicine may raise an eyebrow at the efficacy and reliability of herbal medicine, I have seen it help enough patients of mine that I would never rule out the possibility that it can help ease anxiety.

Of course, given that herbal medicine is less regulated than pharmaceuticals, with less rigorous testing required to bring a product to market, it's a world that requires some research and guidance to navigate. One of the main selling points for herbal medicine is that natural treatments are safer than pharmaceuticals, ideally making them less risky to experiment with. That's often true — for example, I didn't have any reservations about directing Naomi to take a lavender oil supplement, which has no serious negative side effects — but it's worth exercising caution. Just because a substance is natural doesn't mean it's automatically safe. Any herbal preparation should be consumed with medical supervision, whether that means your primary care physician or another health care provider with experience in herbal medicine.

Let's look at some prominent herbal remedies for anxiety and review the research on their effectiveness.

Ashwagandha

Ashwagandha — sometimes referred to as Indian ginseng — is an herb of the Indian Ayurvedic system of medicine, which can be traced back to 6000 BC. According to tradition, the root smells like a horse, and consuming it gives the power of a horse ("ashwa" is the Sanskrit word for horse). Sure enough, in animal studies, ashwagandha has been shown to increase stamina and endurance.[43] More relevant to us, recent studies have shown promising results of the use of ashwagandha to reduce stress and ease anxiety,[44] and a review concluded that all qualifying studies showed ashwagandha was more effective at fighting anxiety than a placebo.[45] The theory is that this herb helps ease stress and anxiety by having a moderating effect on the HPA-axis.[46]

Clinically I've seen this supplement help my patients with anxiety, so it's worth pursuing if other avenues aren't effective. Since ashwagandha naturally has a bitter taste, you may need to try a few different brands before you settle on a clean supplement with a neutral taste and no added sugars.

Berberine

I am asked a lot about berberine, a supplement that went viral and has been called "nature's Ozempic" in the press. From earlier on, you may recall that Ozempic and Wegovy are both prescription medications made popular by their weight-loss effects.

Berberine is a plant supplement obtained from the barberry plant. It is a natural isoquinoline alkaloid obtained from several herbal plants, such as *Berberis Hydrastis canadensis* (goldenseal) and others. Its first documented appearance was in traditional Asian medicine dating back to 3000 BC. Some research has shown that berberine can help lower blood sugar levels and act like a popular prescription medication called metformin, which is widely prescribed for T2D. In addition, a systematic review showed that it reduces insulin resistance. While it's not entirely clear that berberine is a "stand-in" for Ozempic, it has shown some effect on weight loss in a meta-analysis that found a significant reduction body weight, BMI, waist circumference, and C-reactive protein levels associated with berberine intake. It was also thought this may have had an indirect role in helping metabolic disorders. In this way, berberine could potentially help ease anxiety by improving metabolic health.

For anxiety, animal studies have shown some positive impact from berberine. The mechanism to help lower anxiety may be related to its effect on monoamines in the brain stem and the lowering of serotonergic activity. In addition, berberine inhibits glutamate receptors and can lower glutamate, 5-HT (5-hydroxytryptamine) and NE (norepinephrine) levels.

Since we know from chapter 6 that metabolic health is linked to mental health, as more research emerges, berberine may be an option to review with your doctor to help anxiety and/or any weight gain side effect from a psychotropic medication you are prescribed. Again, always discuss any supplement with your doctor before embarking on a trial.

Ginkgo Biloba and Ginseng

Ginkgo biloba and ginseng have been staples of Eastern medicine since ancient times, used for a wide variety of health effects. Ginkgo biloba has been prized for its antimicrobial, anti-inflammatory, and neuroprotective effects.[47] It contains a variety of bioactive compounds, including polyphenols and terpenes, that modulate different neurotransmitter systems. Ginseng is rich in antioxidants and has been used to boost the immune system. While most studies of ginkgo biloba's and ginseng's effects on the brain center on their protection against neurodegeneration, studies have shown that ginkgo biloba improves anxiety symptoms in patients with GAD,[48] and ginseng helps mitigate the effects of stress, with the potential to ease depression and anxiety.[49]

I've seen mixed results in patients who use these two traditional remedies to try to fight anxiety. Still, since they are beneficial in other aspects of health, it may be worth discussing them with your doctor.

Kava

Kava is a plant traditionally used in ceremonial drinks in the Pacific Islands. It has picked up steam throughout the world as an alternative treatment for stress and anxiety. Though it has social effects similar to those of alcohol, kava proponents claim that it eases anxiety and promotes relaxation without any reduction in cognitive abilities.

Some recent medical studies into kava's effectiveness have shown improvement in anxiety symptoms in participants with and without a GAD diagnosis,[50] but others have found insufficient evidence to make a firm conclusion.[51] Given this uncertainty, and possible concerns about effects on the liver (kava has been banned at times in some European countries, though most bans have been lifted), I wouldn't recommend it as a go-to herbal remedy for anxiety.

Passionflower

Passionflower, specifically the species *Passiflora incarnata*, is native to South America, Australia, and Southeast Asia and has been used as an herbal remedy by many different cultures for a variety of different afflictions, including anxiety. It's a rich source of vitamins and minerals, as well as alkaloid and polyphenol bioactives, and several recent studies have sought to prove its effectiveness as a treatment for anxiety and other mental health conditions.

While not every study is in total agreement, a review of recent studies suggests that passionflower has an effect comparable to that of powerful benzodiazepines for quick relief of anxiety. But while those drugs can come with drowsiness and dependence, passionflower has no such side effects, making it an ideal substitute in certain cases.[52] It could be worth a try if you are suffering from acute episodes of anxiety, like panic attacks.

Passionflower is available as a tea, which I often suggest my clients try before they commit to a supplement (see my recipe on page 269 for Passionflower Tisane).

Rhodiola rosea

Rhodiola rosea, also known as roseroot, golden root, or arctic root, grows at high altitudes and in cold climates in Europe and Asia and has been used as an herbal medication in Scandinavia and Russia for centuries. The root of the plant contains adaptogens, substances that help the body adapt to stress, having neuroprotective and antianxiety properties.[53]

Studies have shown that treatment with *Rhodiola rosea* has led to significant improvement in anxiety symptoms among GAD patients[54] and among patients struggling with only mild anxiety.[55] For my patients who aren't seeing strong results from dietary changes, I often recommend trying a *Rhodiola rosea* supplement.

Cannabinoids

Cannabinoids are terpenes found in the cannabis plant. Cannabis is a familiar recreational drug, with ever-growing support as a medical treatment for chronic pain and other conditions. The two most prominent cannabinoids are delta-9-tetrahydrocannabinol (THC) and cannabidiol (CBD). The two compounds have quite different effects, particularly on anxiety. While medical cannabis is sometimes touted as an anxiety treatment, THC, especially in high doses, can actually cause anxiety, leading to feelings of panic and paranoia. CBD has shown promise as an antianxiety treatment.[56]

While there is potential in CBD and other cannabinoids in fighting anxiety, the conversation surrounding them needs to cool down a bit before I'm confident making medical recommendations regarding their use. Too often, discussions about cannabis products end up reflecting either a positive or negative bias, depending on preconceptions about their use. I'm certainly cautious about recommending them—I've spent too much time on call in the busiest Boston emergency rooms treating substance-induced psychoses and related complications to be fully comfortable endorsing cannabis products. However, I remain open to the ongoing scientific research and always feel that science should be served with a dose of humility—we simply don't know everything!

A (BIO)ACTIVE ROLE IN FIGHTING ANXIETY

I want to reiterate that while the bioactives we've discussed in this chapter have the potential to improve anxiety, none of them should be considered a magical cure. Just like all anxiety treatments, they have strengths and limitations, and different people will react to them in different ways. But once you've ensured that you're eating the right balance of macro- and micronutrients, the bioactives in food and supplements can sometimes provide the final boost you need to defeat anxiety.

Now that we know how the component parts of different foods can help relieve anxiety, it's time to develop a balanced, sustainable eating plan full of delicious foods that calm your mind.

CHAPTER TEN

An Antianxiety Shopping Trip

I love grocery shopping. I understand why many people see it as a chore, but it has never felt that way to me. There's something exhilarating about seeing such an abundance of fresh food just waiting to be turned into delicious meals. When left to my own devices, I can spend far too long in a well-stocked produce section, imagining the possibilities. It makes sense that grocery pickup and delivery gained prominence during the COVID-19 pandemic, but I was thrilled when I could don my mask and go back to the store to pick out my own food, brainstorming recipes and browsing foods I've never tried before.

Selecting quality ingredients is one of the best ways to get yourself excited about eating a healthy, antianxiety diet. However, if you're dipping your toes into cooking at home when you're used to eating out, I get that the grocery store can feel a little intimidating—particularly if you're already feeling anxious about other parts of your life. Without an established repertoire of dishes to cook or the confidence to start experimenting, you might feel a little overwhelmed. Rather than picking out whole foods that might require a little more planning and prep work, it can be tempting to reach for prepared and frozen meals—maybe more cost-effective than eating at restaurants, but probably not healthier.

In this chapter, I want to take you on a trip to the grocery store, strolling through the sections to pick out a good mix of healthy, whole foods that can make up the core of your antianxiety diet. Of course, knowing what foods to buy is only one part of the equation; it's equally important to know what foods to avoid. As wonderful as grocery stores can be, they are not going to make responsible food decisions for you; even the "healthiest" grocery store is going to stock plenty of sugary, processed goodies that will worsen your anxiety, so you'll need to be selective about what you put in your cart.

The first step is deciding where to shop. My recommendation is simple: go to whatever grocery store is convenient, comfortable, and in line with your budget and has a decent selection of fresh fruits and vegetables. I sometimes get frustrated by the notion that you must shop at an expensive, specialty grocery store to eat healthy. That's not the case! While specialty grocers like Whole Foods are wonderful, if cost or proximity is a concern, I assure you that you can find healthy food at any standard grocery store or in the grocery section of large chains like Walmart, Target, and Costco.

Of course, in the United States, having access to fresh food is not guaranteed. Many low-income areas are food deserts, with little to no availability of affordable, fresh, healthy food. In 2019, an estimated 23.5 million people lived in a food desert;[1] this has been found to lead to poorer health outcomes across the board, including poorer mental health.[2] If you live in an area where grocery stores are scarce, or struggle to fit healthy food into your budget, I encourage you to seek out local programs that help improve access to healthy food. For instance, in Boston, there are programs run by the city, state, and local nonprofits that improve access to local farmers' markets, incentivize the use of SNAP and EBT on fresh produce, and promote urban farming.

While availability of such programs will vary by city and state, there are many such programs and organizations across the country. Amazon also now accepts SNAP and EBT cards (currently in all states except Alaska) thanks to a new program they developed to provide greater access to fresh food.

PRODUCE

Produce is usually the first thing you see right as you walk in the door of the grocery store. It gives me such a rush of joy to see all those beautiful displays of fruits and vegetables piled high and shining with colorful, delicious nutrition. And as we learned earlier, those vibrant colors aren't just gorgeous to look at; they are an outward expression of the range of powerful nutrients that are all a part of the mosaic of an antianxiety diet.

How Important Is It to Eat Organic?

My patients often ask whether it's worth paying the premium to buy organic produce, grains, meat, and dairy. The answer is somewhat complicated. From a nutritional standpoint, there is evidence to suggest that organic food is healthier in small ways. For example, organic fruits and vegetables do appear to have higher polyphenol content than conventional varieties, and observational studies have shown that eating organic foods has a positive effect on a range of conditions, including metabolic syndrome, cancers, and infertility.[3] Organic meat and dairy tend to have slightly better balances of fats and proteins.[4] Therefore, I do recommend buying organic when possible. But the evidence isn't powerful enough to suggest that you should eat *exclusively* organic food. If buying organic means you can afford less fresh produce, that's not a good trade-off. And being organic doesn't automatically mean being healthy; there are plenty of organic snacks and prepared foods that are highly

---

processed and contain large amounts of unhealthy fats and added sugars. Whether you are buying organic or nonorganic food, make sure you're going for whole foods that are processed as little as possible.

Leafy greens are important for their micronutrient and fiber content and are a great source of polyphenols like lutein, an antioxidant that has shown promise in reducing depression-like symptoms in mice.[5] It's particularly important to eat leafy greens raw in salads, because cooking can remove valuable nutrition. When planning a salad, skip the iceberg lettuce, and instead reach for darker green colors and more complex flavors, like romaine lettuce, arugula, kale, and spinach. If you prefer cooked greens, collard, turnip, and mustard greens are all great sources of vitamins and minerals. And as you get comfortable cooking with greens, you can branch out into even more diverse choices like bok choy, Swiss chard, and dandelion and beet greens.

As we talked about in chapter 8, I absolutely love cruciferous vegetables and view them as a key part of an antianxiety diet thanks to their high levels of micronutrients and helpful phytochemicals. In addition to their potential to fight anxiety, they are rich in sulforaphane, which has been shown to improve serious mental health issues like schizophrenia, help balance hormones, improve immunity, reverse insulin resistance, reduce symptoms of PMS, and support digestion.[6] Several of my favorite leafy greens, like arugula, kale, collard, and turnip greens, are also cruciferous vegetables, but you'll also want to load up the cart with others, like broccoli, Brussels sprouts, cabbage, and cauliflower (see the following table). These can be eaten raw or in a vast range of preparations. If your produce section is particularly well-stocked, you might even find one of my new favorites, the purple sprouting broccoli that is on the cover of this book.

Leafy Greens or Cruciferous Vegetables?

Leafy Greens	Cruciferous Leafy Greens	Cruciferous Vegetables
Beet greens	Arugula	Broccoli
Cilantro	Bok choy	Brussels sprouts
Dandelion greens	Cabbage	Cauliflower
Parsley	Collard greens	Kohlrabi
Romaine lettuce	Kale	Radish
Spinach	Mustard greens	Rutabaga
	Rapini	Turnip
	Swiss chard	
	Turnip greens	
	Watercress	

Other vegetables to keep in mind: red bell peppers are a terrific source of vitamin C. Artichokes are great for dietary fiber, vitamin C, and magnesium. Beets are rich in dietary fiber, folate, nitrates, and antioxidant phytochemicals. Asparagus contains a compound that has been used in traditional Chinese medicine to treat anxiety and has shown promise in modern research as well.[7] Garlic, leeks, and onions provide complementary flavors in food and are rich in prebiotics that help foster a healthy microbiome.

Depending on your grocery store, you may also be able to buy microgreens. Microgreens are the baby versions of many different vegetables, including broccoli, radishes, peas, and leafy greens like arugula. Microgreens have seen an explosion in popularity in recent years because they have a greater concentration of nutrients than their mature versions. While current research on the benefits of microgreens isn't focused directly on anxiety, given their richness in micronutrients and bioactives, there's good reason to try to add them to your diet.[8] Microgreens are often available precut as salad mix, but you can also buy pre-planted trays of live sprouts, which can be trimmed down as needed and then allowed to sprout back up. It's like having a miniature garden in your kitchen!

Fruits are where you can really take advantage of the rich variety of colors for diverse micronutrient and polyphenol content. We've already talked about berries, but I'll emphasize again that they are a delicious sweet treat that is relatively low in sugar and packed with antioxidants and other helpful bioactives. Apples contain the flavonoid quercetin, which has powerful antioxidant and anti-inflammatory effects,[9] and are a great source of fiber. Apples are relatively high in sugar, though, so try to select greener varieties that are a bit less sweet. And make sure you eat the peel, which is where the bulk of the phenolic content is found.

Avocados are a bit different from other fruits and vegetables (they are technically a fruit) in that they have a much higher fat content and a low carb content, leading to a flavor profile that is savory rather than sweet. The fats in avocados are primarily healthy MUFAs that have been shown to decrease oxidation and reduce metabolic risk factors when eaten regularly (and as we'll see shortly, avocado oil is a good alternative to olive oil in high-heat cooking).[10] Avocados are also rich in B vitamins, vitamin E, fiber, and magnesium, so they are a worthy part of your antianxiety diet.

There really isn't much to avoid in the produce section, so I have only a few cautionary notes. Some sweet fruits like watermelon and grapes can add significant sugar to your diet while being relatively low in nutrients. That doesn't mean they need to be totally avoided—I'd much rather you eat a handful of grapes than a cupcake—but think of them as an occasional rather than regular snack. Also be aware that starchy vegetables like potatoes have a high glycemic index and should be eaten only about once a week.

Frozen and Canned Fruits and Vegetables

While fresh fruits and vegetables should be a major part of your diet, they are inherently perishable, which can lead to waste and inconvenience when you aren't able to cook them as soon as you'd hoped.

I do not recommend canned vegetables or fruits. While there are other foods where the convenience and longevity of canned or jarred food is worth a small trade-off in nutrition, that's not the case here. The drop-off in flavor and nutrition between fresh and canned is significant, and preserved fruits and vegetables often include additives like sugar, fruit juice, large amounts of salt, or preservatives. I don't recommend any canned fruits, and no canned vegetables other than canned legumes and canned tomatoes for sauces.

If you do have trouble eating fresh produce before it spoils, frozen options are much better. While there is some variation, most nutrients are well preserved when frozen, and some frozen vegetables actually have more nutrition than fresh, since they are frozen immediately at peak ripeness rather than being picked before they're ripe and then shipped out to stores.[11] In particular, frozen green peas, broccoli, and cauliflower florets are great to have on hand as a quick addition to meals, and frozen berries are ideal for blending with unsweetened yogurt to make a smoothie.

As much as I love the grocery store's produce section, you should also try to visit your local farmers' market for in-season produce. Apart from the fact that you'd be supporting local farmers and eating more sustainably, fruits and vegetables are most nutritious (and delicious) when they're grown to full ripeness and sold as fresh as possible. Small farmers also tend to be passionate about the varieties of plants they grow, so they are more likely to have heirloom varieties that may carry more nutrition than those farmed in larger operations.

MEAT, SOY, EGGS, AND DAIRY

After your cart is loaded with vegetables, your next stop should be the fish counter. As we've discussed at length already, seafood is a wonderful source of healthy protein and is the main source of the omega-3 fatty acids EPA and DHA. Mackerel, herring, tuna, trout, and various shellfish all contain omega-3s, but my favorite is salmon. Salmon is widely available, easy to prepare in many different ways, and so flavorful.

There is some debate over whether you should buy wild-caught or farmed salmon. Pacific salmon, usually wild-caught, is leaner, with more protein and a greater micronutrient content. Atlantic salmon, usually farmed, is around three times fattier, though most of that fat doesn't take the form of helpful omega-3s.[12] Still, both are excellent sources of EPA and DHA. While my preference would be wild-caught, farmed is cheaper and more widely available, so it's still a good choice if it feels more practical.

If you're buying fresh fish, it should smell fairly neutral; if fish smells particularly "fishy," it's probably a bit older. A good seafood counter or fishmonger will cut the fillets you need and ensure they are deboned to make it one step easier for you. If you don't have access to a quality source of fresh fish — or if it's simply not practical for you due to cost or convenience — buying frozen is a convenient and cost-effective option without a significant drop-off in nutrition.[13] Canned seafood is also a good option. Unlike canned vegetables, which are considerably less nutritious than fresh, canned fish and other seafood retain roughly the same nutritional value as fresh, including its omega-3 content. There are even some nutrients, like calcium, that can be more plentiful in canned fish. When choosing canned fish, opt for those canned in water, or higher-quality brands canned in olive oil. Fish canned in other types of vegetable oil is likely to be full of pro-inflammatory PUFAs that can do harm — so as always read the label.

Moving toward the meat counter, we've already discussed changing attitudes about the health effects of saturated fat. In previous eras, I would probably have recommended that you avoid red meat altogether, but given how the research has changed on saturated fat, it's worth including moderate amounts of beef in your diet to capitalize on its excellent source of protein, B vitamins, iron, and other essential nutrients. I do recommend buying sustainably raised grass-fed beef, which is increasingly available in grocery stores. If you don't have good local options, you can order meat from farms that use regenerative agricultural practices.

Sustainable Eating

Patients often ask me how to eat sustainably, especially if they choose to eat meat and dairy. Finding the right balance between health, food preferences, and environmental impact is highly individualized. Medical and environmental science are quite similar in that they are filled with contradictions, misconceptions, and entrenched positions.[14] Most in the scientific community would agree that we're facing colossal challenges to both environmental and personal health, but both are extremely complex systems that defy a one-size-fits-all approach in terms of a correct course of action for each person. Just as I believe that everyone has to determine their own path toward mental and physical health, I believe that everyone should thoughtfully and conscientiously decide how environmental impact should guide what they eat.

For many of my patients, eating sustainably is very much a priority, and I applaud that. And recent studies show that certain eating habits can make a real difference in big environmental challenges like climate change.[15] The cornerstone of these habits is to eat more plant products and fewer animal products, with a focus on whole, unprocessed foods. I trust that sounds familiar to you! Happily, eating to fight anxiety and eating to fight climate change are not mutually exclusive, and in fact, following the recommendations in this book would reduce the environmental footprint of people who are used to a more typical American diet that leans on meat and processed food.

If you do eat meat and dairy, try to find producers who practice regenerative agriculture, which seeks to raise livestock in a sustainable way by following natural grazing patterns rather than feeding confined animals a highly processed diet.[16]

Poultry, like chicken and turkey, is another good source of protein and B vitamins and also provides tryptophan. All types of poultry have roughly the same amount of tryptophan, which is best absorbed by your body if combined with a carbohydrate. Factory-farmed chicken can be more affordable, but it's less nutritious. If possible, I always recommend organic chicken raised without antibiotics.

It's important to remember that even meat eaters should get most of their macronutrients from plant-based sources. My rule of thumb is that two meals a day should be fully plant-based, with meat at only one meal. And some kinds of meat should be avoided entirely. Keep your cart rolling past any type of processed or cured meat, including bacon, sausages, hot dogs, sliced deli meats, and cured meats. Processed meat is often high in added sugar and an excess of unhealthy fat, and the nitrates and nitrites used to preserve meat — even meat labeled "uncured" — have been associated with increased cancer risk.[17]

Meat substitutes like Beyond Meat and Impossible meat are highly processed and designed with taste and texture in mind rather than health, so I would eat these only on occasion rather than treating them as a staple source of protein. Highly processed soy-based meat substitutes like faux-chicken nuggets and veggie dogs should be avoided, too. However, soy, a classic source of plant protein, has shown promise in fighting anxiety.

While soy products like tofu have been eaten for thousands of years in Asian cultures, in the late nineties, the healthiness of soy products was called into question. The issue surrounded the possibility that isoflavones in soy—a type of phytochemical that can mimic the effects of the hormone estrogen in the body—could increase risk of breast cancer and other bad health outcomes.[18] Though this research has been largely debunked—in fact, the isoflavones in soy have been shown to be anti-inflammatory and perhaps even protective against cancer[19]—there is still a bit of a lingering stigma around soy products, particularly among older generations. That's a shame because soy is a great source of protein and has been shown to mitigate anxiety in animal studies.[20] When choosing soy products, opt for edamame, unsweetened soy milk, tofu, and fermented soy products like miso, tempeh, and natto.

Eggs are another good source of protein, as well as vitamin A, B vitamins, choline, and other helpful nutrients. Like soy, eggs had a hit to their reputation toward the end of the twentieth century, since they are a prominent source of dietary cholesterol, long thought to raise cholesterol levels in your blood. However, it turns out that dietary cholesterol doesn't have such a clear effect on blood cholesterol. In recent studies, eggs have not been linked with increased heart disease, serum cholesterol, or high blood pressure.[21] While there is still some debate, there is evidence that moderate consumption of up to one egg per day is safe.[22] If you consume eggs, try to buy pastured eggs, from hens that are allowed to roam free.

Dairy is a good source of protein as well as vitamins and minerals, especially calcium. Try to find grass-fed milk (often marketed as "grassmilk") and dairy, which contain a higher ratio of omega-3s than conventional milk.[23] Fermented dairy products like yogurt, labne, and kefir are good sources of probiotics, helping to promote a healthy microbiome. That's likely a factor in why studies show that yogurt and other fermented dairy products have potential to reduce anxiety and improve stress response.[24] As for cheeses, I recommend hard cheeses like Parmesan, and sheep's milk cheeses like halloumi, both of which are prominent in Mediterranean diets.

When selecting dairy, it's important to ensure that products are minimally processed and don't have added sugar. Processed cheese products like American cheese should be avoided, as should sweetened yogurt (including yogurt packaged with added fruit), chocolate milk, and ice cream. I also recommend avoiding vegetable butter substitutes, which tend to be made with unhealthy omega-6 PUFAs.

If you're plant-based or looking to replace dairy for other reasons, there are a wide variety of alternative milks made from soy, oats, and nuts. I don't object to these in principle, but they are often loaded with added sugar. Make sure to buy unsweetened varieties. It's also possible to make your own alternative milks from scratch (see my recipe for Homemade Hemp Milk on page 267).

LEGUMES, NUTS, SEEDS, AND GRAINS

Beans are an amazing source of plant protein, complex carbs, dietary fiber, and many micronutrients. They should absolutely be a staple of an antianxiety diet. Dried beans are cost-effective and rewarding to cook, allowing you to adjust seasonings and fill your house with delicious aromas. But they take a bit of forethought and planning since they take so long to simmer, and they may not always agree with your schedule. Luckily, there is an almost infinite variety of delicious canned beans, and the nutritional drop-off is minor. Canned beans make a great base for a quick, healthy meal — just be sure to drain them well, rinse off the canning liquid, and buy an organic variety if possible.

The same is true for other legumes like chickpeas and lentils, both of which are used extensively in Indian and Middle Eastern cuisine. Chickpeas hold up well when canned, while lentils cook faster than most other legumes, so they are more commonly bought dried and cooked at home.

Nuts and seeds are nutritional powerhouses, absolutely packed with healthy protein and fat, as well as dietary fiber, vitamins, and minerals. Walnuts, chia seeds, and flaxseeds are good sources of the omega-3 fatty acid ALA. Almonds, pecans, pistachios, cashews, and Brazil nuts contain a wealth of nutrients like vitamin E, magnesium, manganese, and zinc. In addition to snacking on whole nuts, nut butters are a great way to get their nutritional benefits. Just make sure you're eating natural nut butters, with no added sugars or processed vegetable oils.

Most of your carbs should be coming from low-GI sources like legumes. But if you love bread, aim for breads with a lower glycemic index, like fresh-baked sourdough, and eat only one slice once a week or less. Remember that whole wheat bread has roughly the same glycemic index as white bread (though it may be marketed as including more fiber), so it is not to be eaten any more frequently. Once again, most important is to avoid highly processed, mass-produced breads, which often have added sugar and are made with fortified grains. Also avoid bread products that make it easy to over-load on refined flours. For instance, though they may be delicious, bagels tend to be huge bombs of high-glycemic-index carbs. And if you have celiac or any gluten sensitivity, avoid wheat bread entirely.

Pasta is tough because so many of us consider a steaming bowl of spaghetti bolognese or fettucine Alfredo a comforting food we look forward to. But eating a lot of pasta means eating a lot of refined carbs, which we know isn't great for anxiety.

I have three tips if you love pasta.

The first involves an extra culinary step that Italian chefs might balk at: recent research has shown that cooling pasta after it is cooked changes its starch structure in a way that lowers the glycemic index. While it's not all that appealing to eat pasta cold, this positive effect persists even after pasta is reheated.[25] So you might consider cooking your pasta ahead of time, draining it and letting it cool, and then reheating again before you serve it. This trick also works with potatoes—see my recipe for a Baked (and Cooled) Potato on page 250—and other starchy carbs, so try to incorporate it into your cooking as much as possible.

Second, add in more vegetables to your pasta, as this increases fiber and nutrient content. For instance, try my Healthy-ish Mac and Cheese on page 240, which uses cauliflower as the base of the sauce.

Third, a major problem with pasta is that we tend to eat way too much of it in a sitting. Try to plan your meals so that a small portion of pasta is served as an appetizer (as pasta is usually served in Italy) or as a side dish to a main meal that is full of healthy proteins, fats, and vegetables. Like bread, you should try to eat pasta once a week or less.

If you want to be able to eat pasta to your heart's content, you may want to explore pasta substitutes. For instance, I like noodles made from konjak root, which are sold as shirataki or Miracle Noodles. Konjak is a plant native to East and Southeast Asia. It has a starchy root that confers many metabolic benefits, like reducing cholesterol and blood pressure, as well as reducing inflammation and providing prebiotics to encourage good gut health.[26] I recommend thoroughly rinsing these noodles in cool water, then quickly steeping them in boiling water for one to two minutes. Another popular pasta substitute is noodles made from zucchini or spaghetti squash (see my recipe for Spaghetti Squash Noodles with Walnut "Pesto" on page 248).

Rice is an interesting case. White rice has a high glycemic index on par with refined wheat flour, but at the same time, it is a pillar of many healthy, antianxiety cuisines throughout the world, including traditional Indian and Japanese diets. Research shows that when rice is eaten as part of a full meal, its glycemic index can be reduced. In a study of Japanese cuisine, when white rice was combined with vinegar, dairy products, and bean products, its GI dropped by 20–40 percent.[27] Therefore, if eaten in modest quantities alongside other healthy foods, white rice is an option. Brown rice has a nutritional profile similar to that of white rice, so while it's also fine to eat in moderation if you prefer it, it's not as miraculously healthy as it's sometimes marketed to be. Wild rice has more fiber, protein, and antioxidants than white and brown rice, so it can be a good choice. Konjak root is also used to make a rice substitute, sold as shirataki or Miracle Rice. No matter what, think of rice as we did pasta—as a side dish rather than the spotlight of your meal, and no more than once a week.

Oatmeal is an excellent source of fiber, and oats promote good gut health. However, while oatmeal has the potential to be a healthy breakfast, data derived from glucose monitors suggests that oatmeal significantly spikes blood sugar.[28] The type of oats you prepare and the accompaniments you eat them with can exacerbate this effect. First, opt for steel-cut oats, which, though they take a bit longer to cook, are less processed and have a lower glycemic index than traditional rolled or instant oats. Second, when you're eating oatmeal, it's important not to load it up with brown sugar or maple syrup, instead eating it with berries, cinnamon, or nuts. Still, I don't recommend oatmeal as an everyday option, and my patients tend to do best when they eat steel-cut oats for breakfast about once a week.

In my clinic my patients always ask for options, which has taught me to think even more out of the box as a chef. There are many grains that have increased in popularity in recent years—though many of them are traditional staple crops from past eras or other cultures, so it's not as if they've recently been discovered. Whole grains like amaranth, barley, bulgur, spelt, farro, and quinoa tend to be rich in fiber, protein, complex carbs, and micronutrients, and I encourage you to explore them, either in dedicated recipes or by subbing them in for more common grains like rice. Try my made-from-scratch Quinoa Cereal on page 237 for a warming breakfast option that also calms your anxiety.

PANTRY ITEMS: OILS, CONDIMENTS, AND SPICES

Your primary cooking oils should be avocado oil and olive oil, both of which are full of healthy MUFAs and contain a low ratio of omega-6 PUFAs. I prefer to make my salad dressings with extra-virgin olive oil, as it is minimally processed and therefore retains the most micronutrients and bioactives. For higher-temperature cooking, I use avocado oil, since olive oil has a low smoke point and can burn easily. Avocado oil has a slightly lower ratio of MUFAs to PUFAs than olive oil, but it is still much better than most other vegetable oils.[29]

Condiments can really liven up a meal, and some of them are quite good for you, too. In particular, all kinds of pickles — whether pickled cucumbers, pickled peppers, or other pickled vegetables like kimchee and sauerkraut — promote gut health by reinforcing bacterial colonies and feeding the bacteria already living in your gut.[30] I prefer to buy refrigerated fermented foods rather than shelf-stable jarred products, because they require less processing and preservatives and maintain their live active cultures better.

Other condiments with low sugar content are also fine to use, like mustard, low-sodium soy sauce (or tamari if you are gluten-free), and hot sauce. Avoid condiments with large amounts of added sugar, like ketchup, barbecue sauce, hoisin sauce, honey mustard, and some salad dressings.

Herbs and spices not only flavor food; they confer a big boost of micronutrients and bioactives. There's no real downside to using them, other than overseasoning a dish, so I encourage you to experiment with a range of different flavor profiles. For fighting anxiety, I recommend turmeric (with a pinch of black pepper) and saffron (though as we saw in chapter 9, it can be difficult to consume enough of these spices to reach the levels of a supplement), as well as paprika, oregano, rosemary, mint, parsley, and thyme.

BEVERAGES

The most important beverage to drink is water. Hydration is crucial in so many ways, and it's unsurprising that there is some correlation between drinking more water and suffering less depression and anxiety.[31] But there's no reason to buy your water at the grocery store, and tap or filtered water is the more environmentally friendly choice. Claims of health benefits of specialty waters that contain minerals and additives like electrolytes are driven more by marketing than by any real scientific evidence.

If you find that you don't drink enough plain water, seltzer water is an option. Plain seltzer is always the best choice, because it's tough to tell what kind of flavorings companies use. And of course, you should avoid sweetened sodas, whether they contain real sugar, calorie-rich sweeteners like high-fructose corn syrup, or artificial sweeteners. We know that large amounts of sugar can wreck your diet and cause anxiety, but remember that even though your body doesn't process artificial sweeteners into calories, your gut microbiota are still affected. You should be extra careful to avoid energy drinks, which are not only packed with sweeteners but also contain large amounts of caffeine and other compounds that can worsen anxiety. Recent studies have confirmed the commonsense idea that energy drinks are bad for anxiety.[32]

Though I approach caffeine with caution, there is room in an antianxiety diet for moderate amounts of coffee and tea. Tea is the better choice, given its low caffeine content and the helpful polyphenols in both black and green tea. But if you're a coffee drinker, be sure to keep coffee consumption within careful limits. Studies have shown that around 5 cups of coffee can cause panic attacks and raise anxiety in both healthy adults and those who already suffer from panic disorder.[33] While most people don't drink 5 cups of coffee in a sitting, it's not unheard of to drink that much over the course of a day, so if you're used to drinking coffee throughout the day, be cognizant of the fact that you may be drinking more than you think, and try to limit yourself to 2–3 cups.

Alcohol also has a complicated relationship with anxiety disorders. Some anxiety disorders, like social anxiety, may lead to increased alcohol use,[34] but alcohol use can also lead to anxiety.[35] On the other hand, some studies have shown that being a nondrinker is associated with higher odds of having an anxiety disorder.[36] If you do drink alcohol, drink red wine rather than beer or spirits, and no more than 4 glasses a week for women and 6 glasses a week for men. If you choose cocktails, drink what I call clean cocktails, which are not loaded with sugar and added liqueurs and fruit juices. Pay attention to how alcohol makes you feel. If you feel jittery or uneasy, it may be best not to drink at all to better support your anxiety.

SNACKS, SWEETS, AND TREATS

This is the part of the shopping trip where you'll really have to exercise self-control. Snacks are bound to lean toward being unhealthy. They target the part of your brain that wants to gorge on salt, sweetness, and fat. Snack makers nearly always place value on addictiveness and cheap means of production over everything else, so snacks are often made with the lowest-quality ingredients that make you want to eat more of them. It's a dangerous combo, and when I see the aisles overstuffed with bright, glossy packaging of chips, cookies, ice cream, and everything else, I can see why our culture has such trouble resisting these choices.

But resist you must. Keep moving past the chips. Look the other way as you pass the cookies. Don't open the ice cream freezer. Leave the sweetened breakfast cereals on the shelf. Even many foods that are ostensibly healthy, like granola bars, can be packed with added sugars. And snacks made by health food companies, like veggie chips and various organic options, are still highly processed and not much healthier than regular potato chips if you eat the whole bag.

We've already talked about many healthy foods that can double as tasty snacks: a piece of fruit, or vegetables dipped in hummus, fresh salsa, or guacamole. A handful of nuts is an amazing snack, as is plain yogurt. If you need a touch of sweetness with yogurt, I recommend a drop of manuka honey, a variety of honey that is used for medicinal purposes due to its high phenolic content and anti-microbial properties.[37] When it's time for dessert, fruit like berries can scratch the itch, and I always recommend a little dark chocolate.

Buying chocolate can be tricky, since marketing ploys often disguise sugar-laden candy bars as "dark" chocolate. I guide my patients toward extra-dark natural chocolate to maximize brain benefits — ideally chunks of dark chocolate that are not packaged into bars. There have also been recent concerns about the possibility of dark chocolate containing unhealthy levels of cadmium and lead. I recommend doing some research to pick brands that have the lowest levels of these toxic metals, as well as consuming no more than an ounce of chocolate per day, which is more than enough to benefit your health.[38]

A TRIP TO THE GROCERY STORE FOR CALM FOODS

I hope this imaginary trip to the grocery store has you excited about going yourself and filling your cart with delicious, anxiety-preventing foods. But until you've established a regular habit of selecting these antianxiety foods, it can be tricky to remember everything you're supposed to be looking for. I love using acronyms to remember lists of key ingredients. When you're walking around the store or creating your list, remember to include CALM FOODS:

- **Cruciferous vegetables:** Arugula, bok choy, broccoli, Brussels sprouts, cabbage, cauliflower, collard greens, and kale.

- **Anti-inflammatory and antioxidant foods:** Berries, nuts, seeds, and teas, including black, green, and herbal teas.

- **Legumes and leafy greens:** Legumes, including beans, chickpeas, lentils, soybeans; leafy greens, including arugula, chard, romaine lettuce, and spinach.

- **Micronutrients:** Whole, unprocessed foods, including vegetables, legumes, meat, and dairy, are always rich in micronutrients like vitamins A, B_1, B_6, C, and E and minerals like calcium, iron, and magnesium.

- **Fiber and fermented foods:** Fiber, including vegetables, legumes, nuts, and seeds; fermented foods, including kimchi, miso, sauerkraut, and yogurt.

- **Omega-3 fatty acids:** Salmon, nuts, and seeds.

- **Oil:** Extra-virgin olive oil for dressings and drizzles, avocado oil for higher-heat cooking.

- **Dark chocolate:** Extra-dark natural chocolate.

- **Spices and herbs:** Turmeric (with black pepper), saffron, paprika, oregano, rosemary, mint, parsley, and thyme.

Once you get home with your bounty of antianxiety ingredients, you'll be ready to prepare delicious, healthy meals that will put you on the road to calming your mind with food.

PART III: THE PROTOCOL

CHAPTER ELEVEN

The Six Pillars to Calm Your Mind

In 2004, *National Geographic* reporter Dan Buettner set out to discover the places in the world where people live longest, hoping to glean insights into the secrets of longevity. His team's research revealed five places with the highest percentage of residents who live past one hundred years old: Loma Linda, California; Nicoya, Costa Rica; Sardinia, Italy; Ikaria, Greece; and Okinawa, Japan. They deemed these cities the Blue Zones and studied their diets, lifestyles, and philosophies to develop a set of guidelines for long life they called "the Power 9," which includes a range of factors like movement, life outlook, connection with others, and, of course, healthy eating patterns.[1]

The Blue Zones inspired bestselling books and popular TED talks, becoming a foundational study for healthy living. An initiative where aspects of the Power 9 were applied in the city of Albert Lea, Minnesota, led to substantial health benefits to the community, including weight loss and reduced health care costs.[2]

The Blue Zones project was focused on increasing longevity rather than reducing anxiety. However, we know that the biggest impediments to longevity, like chronic inflammation and metabolic disruption, are also major contributors to anxiety. Studies inspired by the Blue Zones have demonstrated how these lifestyle choices can lead to reduced anxiety. For example, during the COVID-19 pandemic, a group of employees at Northern Arizona University participated in a study where they underwent an eight-week program of Blue Zones education, including virtual presentations, cooking demonstrations, and wellness counseling. Even during such a nerve-wracking time, study participants experienced better sleep and decreased depression and anxiety symptoms by the end of the course.[3]

I am confident that living by the Power 9 would help reduce anxiety in many ways; lifestyle factors like increasing movement, reinforcing community, and embracing the power of rest all promote positive mental health effects. But as always, I'm most interested in what we can learn from the Blue Zones' approach to food. Three of the Power 9 apply directly to food, and there are useful lessons in each:

- *Plant Slant:* One Blue Zone, Loma Linda, California, is made up predominantly of vegans, while others include some meat and dairy in their diets. However, *all* of the Blue Zone residents' diets are heavy on plant-based foods, especially beans— an antianxiety superfood due to high levels of fiber, micronutrients, and an ideal balance of low-GI carbohydrates and plant-based protein.

- *The 80 Percent Rule:* This rule comes from the Okinawan mantra "hara hachi bu," which translates to "eat until you are eight parts full." In other words, one should stop eating when 80 percent full. All the Blue Zones residents have a similar practice, often eating the bulk of their food in the morning and at midday, followed by a small meal in the late afternoon or early evening, and then not eating again until the next morning.[4] I certainly concur with this advice and believe in eating everything in moderation.

- *Wine @ 5:* This is the only rule of the Power 9 about which I would offer a note of caution before you adopt it as standard practice. Blue Zones' residents (except for the residents of Loma Linda, California, who abstain for religious reasons) drink moderate amounts of red wine (no more than 4 glasses per week for women and 6 glasses per week for men). We know that red wine is rich in helpful polyphenols and antioxidants that have been shown to have cognitive benefits. However, if you have any trouble at all moderating your drinking, I do not consider wine a must. It is far better to consume no alcohol than too much.

My favorite thing about the Blue Zones study is that it illustrates that there is more than one way to eat a healthy diet, as long as you follow certain dietary principles. While all the Blue Zones populations followed a heavily plant-based diet full of grains, vegetables, and legumes, there was plenty of variation in their individual make-ups. Okinawan diets include little to no dairy, while Sardinian and Greek cuisine is dairy-rich, especially with aged cheeses — though both use goat and sheep milk instead of cow's milk. Sardinian and Costa Rican communities eat more potatoes, though generally in preparations that lowered their glycemic index, like boiling instead of frying.

I would love to see a similar study performed with anxiety in mind, pinpointing the places in the world where people have the calmest, most centered minds. But even without performing a massive, worldwide study, we can use our knowledge of nutritional psychiatry to develop a set of dietary principles that help you fend off anxiety and create calm. Based on the science we explored in part 1 and the wealth of food knowledge we gained in part 2, let's establish Dr. Uma's Six Pillars to Calm Your Mind.

PILLAR 1: EAT WHOLE TO BE WHOLE

The first and most important step to eating an antianxiety diet is to eat whole foods. Use ingredients that are unprocessed, or as minimally processed as possible. Whole grains, legumes, fresh fruits and vegetables, nuts and seeds, and unprocessed meats, eggs, and dairy should make up the bulk of your diet because:

- Whole foods like vegetables, fruits, unprocessed grains, and legumes are good sources of fiber, which is crucial for gut health, fostering a good environment for helpful bacteria to flourish.

- Whole foods are good for metabolic health. Unprocessed carbs are lower in glycemic index, meaning your body processes them more slowly, avoiding spikes in blood sugar. Eating a whole foods diet is strongly associated with improved metabolic factors and a lower risk of heart disease and type 2 diabetes.

- Eating whole foods is like a nutritional cheat code that will help you with every other pillar as well, since processing often saps foods of nutrients and adds unhealthy fats and added sugars.

PILLAR 2: THE CALMING KALEIDOSCOPE PLATE

Variety is valuable. Enhance your vegetable vocabulary by including a large variety of multicolored plants, herbs, and spices in your diet. Your plate should look like a kaleidoscope, filled with vibrant colors that excite your brain and transfix your palate. From the dark green of broccoli and spinach to the bright orange and yellow of carrots and squash, the vibrant reds of raspberries and beets, and the deep blues and purples of blueberries, purple sprouting broccoli, and egg-plant, eating a range of colors helps ensure a healthy supply of nutrients that calm your mind.

- Colorful vegetables and fruits are the primary source of poly-phenols and other bioactives, which have antioxidant and anti-inflammatory properties and promote good health, bring-ing a diversity of microbes to your gut.

- It's not just vegetables and fruits that can bring color, flavor, and anxiety-fighting compounds to your meals. Herbs and spices like saffron, rosemary, turmeric, and basil also provide a boost of bioactives, while enhancing the deliciousness of your meals.

- Eating a wide variety of plants also helps ensure a steady sup-ply of vitamins and minerals that are essential to proper brain function, which is the focus of our next pillar.

PILLAR 3: MAGNIFY MICRONUTRIENTS

Even though we need them in only minuscule quantities, micronu-trients play a huge role in a vast range of body functions, including the processes that keep your brain calm and stable. Since there are so many important vitamins and minerals, eating a wide variety of foods is key, as is identifying any potential gaps in your diet through testing and considering supplementation if necessary. The most important vitamins to help quell anxiety are the B complex, vita-min C, vitamin D, and vitamin E. The most important minerals are calcium, iron, magnesium, and zinc.

- Micronutrients are important for neurotransmitter function, helping produce and regulate mood chemicals like dopamine and serotonin.

- Many micronutrients have antioxidant and anti-inflammatory properties that help protect your brain from long-term decline.

- Test, don't guess: have your doctor run tests to identify micronutrient shortages. If you have any gaps in your micronutrient intake after adjusting your diet, consider taking supplements to make up the shortfall.

PILLAR 4: PRIORITIZE HEALTHY FATS

Your brain is made up of 60 percent fat, and a steady supply of healthy fats is one of the most important factors in keeping it healthy and free of anxiety. But not all fats are created equal. Ensuring that your fat intake comes from the healthiest sources possible is another key to a calm mind.

- Unprocessed oils that are rich in MUFAs like olive oil and avocado oil are anti-inflammatory and promote good gut and metabolic health. They should be your main oils for food preparation, making up the majority of your fat intake.

- Omega-3 PUFAs found in seafood, nuts, and seeds are crucial for reducing anxiety, preventing neuroinflammation, and protecting against neurodegeneration. Eat fatty fish like salmon for EPA and DHA, and nuts and seeds for ALA.

- Though it should not be a major part of your diet, saturated fat from unprocessed meat and full-fat dairy is not as harmful as it was once considered and is acceptable in moderate quantities.

PILLAR 5: AVOID ANXIETY-TRIGGERING FOODS

As you embrace the positive changes you have made to your diet, it's equally important to avoid foods that will undermine your efforts and trigger anxiety. You must be conscientious about avoiding processed, artificial foods, which can promote gut dysbiosis, cause inflammation, and worsen metabolic health.

- High-GI carbohydrates like refined wheat flour, white rice, and other starches spike your blood sugar, which can mean a burst of energy followed by a crash, a boom-and-bust cycle that is correlated with anxiety.

- Added sugars are high-GI foods and have little to no nutritional benefit. While you will get natural sugars from fruits and vegetables, added sugars should be kept to a minimum. And don't just replace them with artificial sweeteners—while they may not pack the same calories as sugar, they can just as easily lead to gut dysbiosis and worsen anxiety.

- Omega-6 PUFAs in vegetable oils like safflower, soybean, and sunflower oil have an unearned reputation for being healthy, but they are pro-inflammatory, and I recommend avoiding them as much as possible. Be particularly careful to eliminate packaged snacks and deep-fried foods and fast food, which are loaded with unhealthy fats, including pro-inflammatory PUFAs and sometimes trans fats.

PILLAR 6: FIND CONSISTENCY AND BALANCE

Our minds are with us for the rest of our lives. To quell anxiety and achieve calm in the long term and optimize our mental health in a lasting way, it's important to create sustainable dietary and lifestyle changes rather than falling into quick fixes and miracle diets. The best diet for your brain is one that is packed with healthy food, but also one that you can *enjoy*. Eating is about powering your body but also about the pleasure that comes from a delicious meal.

- Build your diet around healthy foods that you love. Whether they're central to your culture's cuisine or simply favorite foods that make you feel calm and secure, we all have foods that are important to us. Rather than forcing yourself to acclimate to a whole new nutrition plan, pursue healthy foods that fit the flavor profiles and ways of eating that *you* love by applying these pillars to your favorite types of food.

- Use your body intelligence to gauge how dietary changes affect your anxiety. If you feel cranky, irritable, hungry, and jumpy after eating certain foods, try cutting them out of your diet. If something doesn't make you feel good after eating it, it's probably not good for you.

- If you eat unhealthy food occasionally, be kind to yourself. I sometimes have patients whose anxiety is worsened by the guilt of eating cake at a child's birthday or a plate of French fries when out with friends. But if you're otherwise succeeding at making healthy eating a habit, you don't need to beat yourself up about occasional deviations from the plan.

THE POWER OF THE PILLARS

Just as following the Power 9 sets a blueprint for longevity, following the Six Pillars is a revolutionary way to control your anxiety through the food you eat. Rather than thinking of anxiety as an above-the-neck problem, making the gut-brain connection work to calm your anxiety is key. If you already follow healthy eating patterns, don't struggle with your weight, and are in safe ranges in metabolic indicators like blood pressure and cholesterol, making changes could be as simple as identifying a set of antianxiety swaps to your current food choices, like switching to olive oil or avocado oil instead of using other types of vegetable oil, adding a greater variety of vegetables to your repertoire, or cutting out added sugars. Eating to improve your mental health isn't an all-or-nothing proposition, and every small choice you make to bring your eating habits closer to the Six Pillars can help reduce your anxiety.

However, if you or your doctor feels you're in need of a deeper dietary reset, I recommend starting from square one to reimagine the way you eat, leaning on the power of the Six Pillars to help determine a new way to guide you toward the knowledge and confidence to plan, cook, and eat healthy meals that will calm your mind. In the next two chapters, we will explore how to do just that.

CHAPTER TWELVE

Building Your Antianxiety Eating Plan

When my patients first come into my clinic, they are often confused about what to eat. It's not hard to see why. The loudest voices in the diet wars are constantly competing to have the newest advice about the exact right way to eat, churning out a steady stream of content that promises a one-size-fits-all solution. When I tell my patients there is no magic diet or secret sauce that will immediately and definitively cure anxiety forever, I understand why they might feel a little disappointed. There is comfort in the idea of a set of instructions that fix a problem with no threat of uncertainty.

But while no diet is a magic bullet for every single person, there is value in some of the popular diets that are buzzed about in the media. In fact, the two diets my patients ask about most are the same two that have the best grounding in science and research: the Mediterranean diet and the ketogenic diet. While the principles of the two diets are quite different, they can both be shaped around the Six Pillars to form the basis of a personalized antianxiety eating plan that's right for you. In this chapter, we'll consider the strengths and weaknesses of each diet and break down ways to fit them more snugly into the framework of our Six Pillars. We'll also go over some good eating practices to implement no matter what plan you choose to follow.

THE BEST PLACE TO START FOR MOST PEOPLE: THE MEDITERRANEAN DIET

The Mediterranean diet is based on the traditional diets of cultures located around the Mediterranean Sea, including Greece, Italy, southern France, Spain, and parts of the Middle East—including the Blue Zones of Sardinia, Italy, and Ikaria, Greece. In the mid-1950s, scientist Ancel Keys sought to figure out why the poor population of southern Italy was so much healthier than the much wealthier population of New York City. His initial curiosity led to the famous Seven Countries Study, which studied the diets of the United States, Finland, Yugoslavia, Japan, the Netherlands, Italy, and Greece. The Seven Countries Study is acknowledged as the first major study to link diet with cardiovascular disease, and it found that diets from the Mediterranean region were the most heart-healthy.[1]

In the 1960s, this research resulted in the development of a diet inspired by Mediterranean cultures, heavy in olive oil, fruit, vegetables, legumes, whole grains, and fish. While the Mediterranean diet has been refined and modified over the years, it is still very much a touchstone of good health. Though long-term studies of complex diets are notoriously difficult to perform due to extended time frames and endless dietary variables, the Mediterranean diet's anti-inflammatory properties and positive effects on cardiovascular and metabolic health have been confirmed many times over. In just one example, a 2020 review found that following the Mediterranean diet led to improved metabolic health in those suffering from type 2 diabetes, as well as a whopping 30 percent reduction in heart attack and other major cardiovascular events.[2] It also leads to a more diverse gut microbiome compared to the standard American diet.[3]

The foods that make up the Mediterranean diet align well with the Six Pillars. It is built around whole foods and includes a wide variety of vegetables, micronutrients, and healthy fats, without including large amounts of anxiety-inducing red flags like added sugars and other high-glycemic-index carbs. As with all associations between diet and mental health, the Mediterranean diet's effect on conditions like anxiety have only been recently studied in earnest. Unsurprisingly, there are strong indications that the Mediterranean diet is beneficial for depression and anxiety.[4] One long-term Swedish study followed almost one hundred thousand Swedish women for twenty years, tracking their adherence to the diet. Results showed that participants who had higher adherence to the Mediterranean diet were less likely to be diagnosed with depression, especially serious depression.[5] While there hasn't been a similar long-term study on anxiety specifically, since these conditions are so closely linked, I feel strongly that it is a good choice for reducing anxiety, too.

In other words, in theory, faithfully following a Mediterranean diet plan is a viable strategy for eating all the foods necessary for a calm mind. In fact, the Mediterranean diet probably is the closest we have gotten to the magical one-size-fits-all diet for general health, so it makes sense that it is so commonly recommended by doctors and dietitians, including myself.

However, it's important to acknowledge the Mediterranean diet's weakness: a lack of flexibility. While its components might be universally healthy, that doesn't mean every person will find it easy to follow and enjoy. Its reliance on seafood and dairy makes it difficult for vegetarians and vegans to follow faithfully. Moreover, a diet based heavily on traditional Mediterranean foods and flavors is simply not going to be a perfect fit for everyone. After a lecture on the benefits of the Mediterranean diet, one of my very smart med students in the Division of Nutrition at Harvard asked me why the Mediterranean diet is so universally recommended, given that many cultures eat very different food. Being Asian, she wasn't interested in revamping her diet around Mediterranean principles, nor did she feel comfortable suggesting that her patients from a diverse range of cultures do so. That made me realize that I feel the same way; though there are many traditional Mediterranean foods and dishes that I love, I would never want to be cut off from the South Asian cuisine I grew up with, or any other world cuisine for that matter.

Sure enough, when I see my patients struggle with the Mediterranean diet, it's often because of conflicts with Pillar 6: Find Consistency and Balance. If the Mediterranean diet doesn't match up with your preferences due to cultural reasons, dietary restrictions, or personal taste, it can be difficult to stick with it consistently. And even if you don't have a strong connection to your own cultural food tradition, you want to make sure you're taking advantage of the ability to eat healthy foods from around the globe—for instance, the avocados and black beans of Latin American cuisine, the nori and miso of East Asian cuisines, and the dal and spices of South Asian cuisines. All of those are excellent foods to fight anxiety, so there's no reason to leave them out simply because they aren't traditional Mediterranean foods.

Happily, there are many options for expanding the confines of the Mediterranean diet to incorporate different foods, while still following the guidance of the Six Pillars. For instance, researchers and recipe developers have explored hybrid MediterrAsian diets that seek to combine the fundamentals of the Mediterranean diet with foods from traditional Asian diets, providing room for different flavors as well as the bioactives in soy, seaweed, green tea, and turmeric, which can enhance the effects of the traditional Mediterranean diet.[6] In my own cooking and clinical work, I've had great success in adding healthy South Asian foods, Korean and Japanese flavors, and other diverse twists to the basics of the Mediterranean diet—which are reflected in the recipes in this book.

To see that in action, let's break down the specifics of an eating plan that synthesizes the Mediterranean diet with a variety of foods and flavors from around the world, all while fitting the framework of the Six Pillars. Since the strengths of the Mediterranean diet are so universal, this Mediterranean-inspired eating plan is what I would first recommend to someone who is just starting the journey to calming their mind with food—and it is the inspiration for the recipes in chapter 14.

THE MEDITERRANEAN-INSPIRED ANTIANXIETY EATING PLAN

Eat Daily:

These daily foods will form the foundation of your antianxiety diet, providing you with a good balance of macronutrients, micronutrients, healthy fats, and fiber.

- Eat at least two different fresh vegetables with every main meal, for a total of 6–8 servings of vegetables daily. Prioritize 1 cup servings of raw, leafy greens (spinach, arugula, romaine) and ½ cup servings of lightly cooked cruciferous vegetables (broccoli, Brussels sprouts, cauliflower), mixing in brightly colored vegetables like bell peppers, tomatoes, carrots, cucumbers, and zucchini, as well as garlic, leeks, and onions.

- Eat 2 servings of fruit daily, either as part of a meal or as a snack or dessert. My favorite single servings of fruit are ¼ cup blueberries; ¼ cup combination of raspberries, blackberries, and strawberries; a small to medium apple; a clementine; or a small orange.

- Daily protein requirements can be calculated using the dietary reference intakes calculator from the USDA (https://www.nal.usda.gov/human-nutrition-and-food-safety/dri-calculator), but you should consult with your doctor, as protein requirements can change with different medical conditions. The best everyday sources of protein are plant-based, for example, 4 ounces organic, non-GMO tofu (about 9 grams of protein); ½ cup lentils (about 9 grams of protein); ½ cup kidney, black, navy, or cannellini beans (about 8 grams of protein); or ½ cup chickpeas (about 6 grams of protein).

- If you choose to eat animal protein, try to keep two meals per day plant-based, and then eat 1 serving of meat, fish, poultry, or eggs at your third meal. Options are 3–4 ounces wild-caught salmon (about 30 grams of protein), 4–5 ounces pasture-raised chicken or turkey (about 30 grams of protein), 4 ounces grass-fed beef (about 33 grams of protein), or 1–2 pasture-raised eggs (12 grams of protein).

- Extra-virgin olive oil: 1–2 tablespoons in salad dressings and other low-heat uses; avocado oil for higher-heat cooking.

- Nuts (walnuts, pecans, almonds): about ¼ cup.

- Seeds (flaxseeds, chia seeds, hemp seeds): about ¼ cup.

- Fermented foods (pickles, kimchi, sauerkraut): ¼ cup

- Tea (lavender, passionflower, chamomile, golden chai): 1–2 cups.

Eat a Few Times per Week:

These foods shouldn't be eaten every day, but they are still good components of an antianxiety diet and can be eaten two to four times per week.

Dairy, preferably grass-fed: ½ cup milk, cottage cheese, or plain yogurt; or 1 ounce Parmesan cheese (plant-based milk, yogurt, and homemade cheese substitutes all work for those who prefer a plant-based diet).

Avocado: ¼ medium-size avocado.

Chocolate: 1½ ounces extra-dark chocolate as a brain-healthy post-meal treat.

Eat No More than Three to Four Times Per Month:

While these foods are not staples, they can be eaten in moderate portions once a week or less. Pay attention to your body intelligence after eating these foods. If you feel nervous, jittery, or cranky after eating starches or grains, cut them out entirely.

Bread and pasta made from wheat flour: 1 slice of bread (preferably sourdough), or 2 ounces dried pasta (cooked and thoroughly cooled before reheating to eat).

White or brown rice: ½ cup or less cooked rice.

Potatoes and sweet potatoes: 1 medium-size potato, baked, boiled, or roasted rather than fried (cooked and thoroughly cooled before reheating to eat).

Meat substitutes: 1 serving as indicated on packaging.

Always Avoid:

These foods and beverages are ubiquitous and tempting, but it's important to avoid them as much as possible, as all can be major anxiety triggers.

- Processed and packaged foods like breakfast cereals, granola bars, chips, and crackers

- Processed meats and cheeses, including sliced deli meat and American cheese

- Sweets like cookies, cakes, and candy, including those sweetened with artificial sweeteners

- Sweet drinks, including soda (regular and diet), fruit juice, energy drinks, and sports drinks

A Sample Meal Plan

Turning those guidelines into a set of real-life meals is the fun part. Here is a sample seven-day meal plan that follows the Six Pillars and combines the healthy foods of the Mediterranean diet with foods and flavors from around the world.

Snacks (choose 1–2 per day):

- 2 tablespoons Brain-Food Granola (page 236) with yogurt or cottage cheese

- ¼ cup blueberries or other mixed berries

- ½ cup organic grassmilk cottage cheese with a sprinkle of cinnamon

- ½ cup grassmilk dairy or nondairy yogurt with cinnamon or plain applesauce and a drop of manuka honey

- Sliced Fuji apple with 1 ounce Parmesan cheese

- 2 tablespoons hummus with celery sticks

Monday

- Breakfast: Basil Seed Pudding (page 233) with blueberries and almonds

- Lunch: Korean-Inspired Shrimp (page 243) with a side of Pan-Seared Purple Sprouting Broccoli (page 260)

- Dinner: Show-Stopping Roasted Head of Broccoli (page 247) with steamed garlicky spinach

Tuesday

- Breakfast: Two-egg omelet or Chickpea Scramble (page 235) with spinach, scallions, and mushrooms

- Lunch: Dr. Uma's Crunchy Kaleidoscope Salad (page 256) topped with Shiitake Bacon (page 261)

- Dinner: Sambar (Dal) (page 245) with vegetables; Go-To Calm Green Salad (page 255) with veggies, nuts, and seeds

Wednesday

- Breakfast: Yogurt (dairy or nondairy) and berries with cinnamon and a touch of manuka honey

- Lunch: Korean-Indian Baked Chicken (page 242) with Spicy Crunchy Cucumber Salad (page 262); or substitute non-GMO organic tofu or Burmese Chickpea Tofu (page 238) for chicken

- Dinner: Mixed salad with shredded red cabbage, carrots, sliced cucumbers, and grape tomatoes; and Baked (and Cooled) Potato (page 250) with chopped scallions, crème fraîche, and grated Parmesan cheese

Thursday

- Breakfast: Quinoa Cereal (page 237) topped with berries

- Lunch: Healthy-ish Mac and Cheese (page 240) with a side green salad

- Dinner: Spaghetti Squash Noodles with Walnut "Pesto" (page 248), or add sautéed ground turkey; and chopped vegetables with Crispy Tikka Masala Tofu (page 239)

Friday

- Breakfast: Chopped avocado with tomatoes and lettuce on sourdough toast, and ¼ cup blueberries

- Lunch: 6 ounces Burmese Chickpea Tofu (page 238) stir-fried with mixed veggies and seasoned konjak Miracle Rice

- Dinner: Cauliflower seasoned with South Asian tikka masala spice blend—just omit the tofu from the recipe on page 239—with air-fried Crispy MediterrAsian Okra Fries (page 253) and arugula salad

Saturday

- Breakfast: Tofu, spinach, and red pepper scramble (substitute 2 pastured eggs instead of tofu, if desired); and sliced strawberries

- Lunch: MediterrAsian-Inspired Eggplant (page 257) with Miso-Infused Cipollini Onions and Green Beans (page 259)

- Dinner: Creamy Cannellini Bean and Greens Soup (page 251), baby bok choy, and romaine salad

Sunday

- Breakfast: Dr. Uma's Cherry CALM Smoothie (page 266)

- Lunch: Curried Cauliflower and Coconut Soup (page 252) with microgreens; side of roasted crispy chickpeas

- Dinner: Konjak Miracle Noodles with peanut sauce and shaved veggies, or add chopped grilled chicken, tofu, chickpeas, or beef

That's a week's worth of meals to keep your mind calm and your tastebuds engaged, following the Six Pillars and the basics of the Mediterranean diet without being tied down to the foods and flavors of a single region.

A LOW-CARB OPTION: CLEAN KETO

Many of my patients are interested in low-carb diets, attracted by their reputation for helping people lose weight. In particular, I'm often asked about the ketogenic diet, a low-carb, high-fat diet that has taken the diet world by storm. While I don't think the restrictiveness of the keto diet is necessary for most people, in situations where a patient's anxiety doesn't respond to a Mediterranean-based eating plan, or weight loss is a priority, there is enough compelling evidence on keto's benefits to mental health that I believe it's worth a try—at least as long as it is adapted to uphold our Six Pillars.

Given its sudden explosion in popularity, you might think the ketogenic diet was a recent invention. But in fact, it was developed as a treatment for epilepsy in the 1920s, with roots that date back to ancient times. The goal of the keto diet is to essentially mimic fasting, tricking your body into thinking it's not getting enough sustenance, convincing it to burn fat for fuel. When you reduce your levels of carbohydrates to less than 15 percent of your caloric intake, your body doesn't have its usual flow of glucose to power the processes of life. In the absence of its favorite fuel, it turns to burning fat for energy. When controlled through careful dieting, this begins a process called nutritional ketosis (a state of uncontrolled ketosis is called ketoacidosis, which can be harmful and even life-threatening). Your liver creates compounds called ketones, which substitute for glucose as the power source for your brain and body. If you weren't eating at all, ketosis wouldn't be sustainable; your fat reserves would eventually be exhausted, and you would be in major trouble. However, if you followed the keto diet, you'd be significantly lowering carbs but constantly ingesting calories from fat (and to a lesser degree protein), which would allow your body to sustain nutritional ketosis indefinitely. Essentially, you'd be switching your body's fuel source from glucose to fat.

The fat-burning process of nutritional ketosis is why the keto diet is so effective at promoting weight loss. However, we now also have a greater understanding of its effects on the brain and its possibilities for reducing anxiety.[7] There is evidence that the keto diet helps reduce inflammation, as well as limiting oxidative stress.[8] The theory is that the metabolism of ketones results in less harmful free radicals than glucose metabolism, and this lowers your risk of chronic inflammation.

Studies of the keto diet's impact on mental health have been encouraging: one comprehensive review into the effects of the keto diet on a range of psychiatric conditions, including depression, bipolar disorder, and schizophrenia (unfortunately, anxiety was not included), found that every single study showed positive mental health effects.[9] Another study found that the diet significantly improved depression and anxiety in patients with Parkinson's disease.[10] Still, our understanding of the keto diet's long-term effects on mental and physical health are relative unknowns given how recently it has risen to prominence. For instance, research into how the keto diet affects the gut microbiome has been mixed, with some studies showing that it enhances diversity of gut bacteria and others showing that it impedes it.[11]

Since so much of a high-fat diet flies in the face of traditional dietary advice, I can see why many health practitioners have been cautious about recommending it. That being said, I am excited about what new research will show, and I do think the keto diet is here to stay as a powerful short-term dietary tool to help anxiety as needed.

CLEANING UP THE KETO DIET

Unlike the Mediterranean diet, keto diets aren't defined by specific foods, instead focusing on a specific breakdown of macronutrients. For example, a typical keto diet may specify that you eat 55–60 percent of calories from fat, 30–35 percent of calories from protein, and 5–10 percent of calories from carbs.[12] But keto diet plans don't always specify the sources of those macronutrients, which can lead unaware dieters to unhealthy food choices — particularly unhealthy fats, like pro-inflammatory omega-6 PUFAs. To complicate matters, many food producers have capitalized on the rise of keto diets to market packaged foods as keto-friendly, even though they are highly processed and often include artificial sweeteners.

Therefore, when my patients are curious about trying the keto diet, I recommend a variation called "clean keto," which strives to meet the dietary components of the keto diet while also emphasizing healthy food. As with the Mediterranean diet, fats should largely come from olive oil, oily fish, avocados, nuts, and egg yolks. Protein comes from dairy, unprocessed meat, and eggs. The small amount of carbs comes from complex, low-glycemic sources like asparagus, spinach, mushrooms, lettuce, and tomatoes, which also contain dietary fiber.

Adapting our Mediterranean-inspired eating plan to fit a clean keto mold requires a number of changes to increase fat consumption and restrict carbs.

- The biggest omission from a Mediterranean-inspired diet is legumes. Beans, chickpeas, and lentils are all too carb-heavy to be included on a keto diet. However, most other protein sources, like tofu, poultry, meat, and seafood are allowed.

- A wide variety of vegetables is still crucial on a clean keto diet — especially since you're cutting out many other good sources of dietary fiber like beans. Leafy greens, cruciferous vegetables, asparagus, bell peppers, mushrooms, onions, garlic, and other low-carb vegetables are allowed. However, you will need to totally avoid starchy vegetables like potatoes, sweet potatoes, corn, beets, and peas.

- Fruits are not allowed. Some keto diets do allow for small amounts of berries, but no other fruits. Increasing intake of healthy fats means consuming more olive oil, nuts, seeds, and avocados. While plant-based fats are always important to include, keto diets are easier if you eat animal fats, especially full-fat dairy and omega-3 fats from salmon and other seafood.

- Grains like wheat and oats should be completely avoided. No bread or pasta.

Keto is not for everyone, and I understand that many are leery of the fad-diet messaging surrounding it and skeptical that eating large amounts of fat is the key to good health — and there are certainly medical researchers who have called into question the long-term wisdom of low-carb diets.[13] Because of these concerns, and because of the level of dedication it takes to stick to a keto diet, in my clinic I reserve the clean keto plan for individuals who have tried a more general Mediterranean-style diet and continue to struggle with both anxiety and weight gain. As they begin to follow clean keto, they are carefully assessed during a trial period to ensure that they can handle the food restrictions while still managing to properly nourish themselves.

While there is reason for caution, if your anxiety hasn't responded to other, less radical dietary interventions, I encourage you to work with a dietary practitioner to develop a plan for a clean keto diet. It could potentially have a major effect on your mental health.

INTERMITTENT FASTING

Along with the keto diet, another rising star in the nutritional world is the concept of intermittent fasting, a dietary practice that has gained a fervent following in recent years for its potential to promote weight loss and improve metabolic health. The basic idea of intermittent fasting is that you eat only during certain windows of time. While there are many variations of intermittent fasting, they all involve eating only in planned intervals, punctuated by periods of fasting where you eat very little or nothing at all. For example, a daily intermittent fasting plan might involve eating for eight hours of the day, then fasting for the following sixteen hours. Another popular approach is the 5:2 plan, where you eat normally five days a week while eating only minimal calories on the other two.

The science on intermittent fasting is not ironclad at this point, but there is promising research that suggests it can be a valuable tool for weight loss, metabolic health, and leptin function, all of which we know can be beneficial for anxiety.[14] There has also been research into the effects of intermittent fasting on anxiety directly, largely stemming from studies surrounding the Islamic holiday of Ramadan, where adherents ritually fast from dawn to dusk. Though religious fasting stems from a different mindset than fasting for general health, it's still promising to see that these studies show a positive effect on depression and anxiety.[15]

There is also evidence that intermittent fasting is beneficial to the diversity of your gut microbiome. Gut microbiota composition fluctuates cyclically throughout the day, and certain eating patterns, like eating close to bedtime, can disrupt these fluctuations, leading to a reduction in microbiome diversity. Intermittent fasting has been shown to normalize patterns in your microbiome and lead to greater diversity, which in turn can help reduce anxiety.[16]

In the absence of more direct research tying intermittent fasting to a reduction in anxiety, it's not something I recommend to every one of my patients. But if a patient is suffering from anxiety and metabolic disruption, it can provide an additional lever to pull alongside changes to diet. If you're curious about trying intermittent fasting, it's worth speaking to a health practitioner to help you develop a plan. While there are several safe methods of intermittent fasting, restricting calories for long periods can be dangerous, especially for people with conditions like diabetes, so it's important to get professional guidance.

GOOD EATING PRACTICES

In addition to choosing foods and planning meals based on the Six Pillars, the final piece of your antianxiety diet is establishing good eating practices to help ensure that meals are a time of calm and free of stress. First, let's return to the wisdom of the Blue Zones, to think about some ways in which the rules of the Power 9 that don't directly pertain to food can be viewed through a dietary lens.

- *Community:* A sense of belonging and a commitment to family and other loved ones are central focuses of the Power 9. For us, this means finding a caring and comfortable community to eat with. That will look different for everyone! For some, it may be the classic family dinner. For others it may be a larger group of people in a church or community group who come together to celebrate food. For still others it may mean joining a friend on video chat for a shared meal, one of the positives that modern technology enabled during the COVID-19 pandemic, one that will remain useful in our increasingly far-flung society.

- *Downshifting:* Residents of the Blue Zones reduce stress by finding opportunities to step away from the pressures of the day. I encourage you to use mealtimes as a chance for respite and relaxation. Sit down at the table rather than eating on the run. Turn off cell phones and laptops, and try not to eat in front of the TV.

- *Eating with purpose:* One of the Power 9 is to live with purpose, and I believe it's important to eat with purpose, too. Acknowledge that you are eating to nourish your body and brain to defeat anxiety. Be mindful about your food. Chew thoughtfully. Pay attention to flavor. Don't feel guilt or regret about the food you eat. Enjoy every bite from the first to the last.

Looking beyond the Power 9, let's meet two last patients of mine who needed to reset their eating practices before they could reap the benefits of an antianxiety diet.

THE DANGERS OF OVER-RESTRICTION

While I believe strongly in practicing concepts like hara hachi bu to avoid overeating, it's also important to be aware that anxiety can push some people in the opposite direction, leading to overly restrictive eating practices that can leave them undernourished and overlap with other serious mental health concerns like eating disorders.

Annie was in her second year of college when she came to me with severe anxiety about her weight and appearance. Her anxious feelings were so powerful that she was avoiding all social situations because she was ashamed of how she looked. I was careful not to register surprise when she told me she had always struggled to lose weight, but it was very clear she wasn't overweight. If anything, she looked significantly *under*weight. It seemed likely that Annie was suffering from body dysmorphic disorder, a psychiatric condition that was causing her to obsess about perceived flaws in her body that weren't evident to anyone else.[17]

When we discussed what she ate, she assured me she ate very clean: fresh vegetables, chicken breast, and occasionally salmon, with no red meat and no added sugar. That sounded like a conventionally healthy diet, but as we talked further it became clear that she was eating small portions, fasting often, and rejecting many types of whole, unprocessed foods. Annie's body dysmorphia was being compounded by a case of orthorexia nervosa, a condition in which people are obsessed with the quality of their food and overdo it on restrictive behaviors.[18]

Annie's consultation put me on high alert. In my clinic, I am unable to work with patients who have active eating disorders—whether they are suffering from a highly restrictive anorexic-type disorder or binge eating. Patients with eating disorders need close monitoring of both their physical health (lab monitoring of hydration levels and hypoglycemia, for example) and their emotional health, as eating disorders can often lead to self-harm or suicide.[19] People struggling with eating disorders often need psychiatric hospitalizations, and some may need a residential treatment program specializing in eating disorders.

After spending time with Annie and speaking with her about her underlying emotions surrounding food, I assessed that her restrictive eating was not yet advanced enough to pose an immediate threat to her physical health. And though she was deeply anxious, she was not at risk of harming herself. Instead of referring her to more intensive care, I decided to help her develop a personalized nutritional psychiatry treatment plan. My first step was bringing in two other team members: Alex, a nutrition coach, and an eating disorders counselor to help her work through the deeper issues that were surfacing through her food behaviors.

I started her on an SSRI to help manage her anxiety, and she spoke twice weekly to her counselor to improve and heal her relationship with food. Alex worked alongside Annie and me, helping to plan shopping trips where they would touch, feel, and explore more foods to add to her diet. Alex would ask Annie to write out a shopping list for the week, then we'd work together to gently encourage her to include more than the foods she was eating. We helped her understand the nutritious value of an expanded whole foods diet. We did not pay attention to weight or a scale. Noticing that her body dysmorphic disorder had kept her hiding under bulky clothes, when she was ready, we suggested she plan a shopping trip with a girlfriend to buy some new clothes and indulge in a hair and makeup session. Incrementally, she gained confidence and felt emotionally stronger until she was able to eat a wider range of foods, reach a healthy weight, and gain perspective on her body dysmorphia.

As I saw with Annie, orthorexia nervosa is recalcitrant and very often correlated with anxiety and low self-esteem,[20] so it's something I keep a close watch for in my patients as we redesign their diets toward healthier food. As important as it is to eat unprocessed, healthy food, it is equally important to maintain proper perspective on setting realistic goals and understanding that it's possible to take an obsession with healthy eating too far. Even patients who don't approach full-blown orthorexia nervosa can fall into the trap of letting the perfect be the enemy of the good, getting frustrated when they stray from their eating plan while traveling, celebrating, or participating in work functions. That's exacerbated by the constant pressure and flood of (often incorrect) advice from social media. It's always important to remember that your body is resilient and that no one meal is going to make or break your quest to escape anxiety. That's why I recommend following overarching guidelines like the Six Pillars, rather than trying to account for each calorie; it's far more important to change eating habits in a way that is sustainable for your lifestyle rather than chasing perfect adherence to a specific plan.

REDEFINING A DIFFICULT RELATIONSHIP WITH FOOD

For patients who come to me with a difficult relationship with food—whether a history of unsuccessful dieting for weight loss, a tendency toward binge eating, or over-restrictive eating like Annie—I often find that helping guide them to healthier foods and developing a personalized nutritional psychiatry meal plan is only one part of the process. There is also work to be done to reframe how they think about eating, opening the door to allow food to calm their minds.

Kayu was a Japanese woman who had immigrated to the United States in her early thirties. In Japan, she had eaten a traditional

Japanese diet full of seafood and vegetables, which meshed very well with the Six Pillars, and she told me that she'd generally felt calm and focused in her work as a hairdresser. When she moved to the United States, her habits changed. She was nervous about integrating into American culture, so she ate what her friends ate, often binging on fried foods and pizza. She still ate Japanese food frequently but found herself gravitating toward Americanized Japanese food that she had never eaten in Japan, like fried chicken wings and tempura, all served with copious amounts of rice.

When she came to see me, Kayu was in such a heightened state that she was barely able to get a word out. She told me that her hands were shaking at work — not something anyone wants but particularly bad for a hairdresser — and that after a significant weight gain, she hardly recognized herself. Her stress and anxiety about her weight gain led her to seek out more comfort food. She realized her new eating patterns were unhealthy, but she felt like she couldn't change them, since food had become the only thing that could calm her down. Most troublingly, she told me she had started to hate herself.

I empathized with Kayu and explained to her that she was not alone. Many immigrants to new countries go through a process called dietary acculturation, changing their diets dramatically in an attempt to fit into a new culture. A recent review looked at dietary acculturation in East Asian immigrants moving to Western countries, and the diet-related disorders that can arise, including increased risk of diabetes and cardiovascular disease.[21]

I recognized that Kayu's biggest problem wasn't knowing what to eat — she now knew that her traditional Japanese diet was intertwined with her mental health — it was that she needed to redefine her relationship with eating on a deeper level.

When I first started to talk to her about ways to change her relationship with food, she wasn't interested. She told me that the body positivity movement irked her and that all she wanted was help losing weight and fixing her mood so that she could get her old life back. I explained that while I could certainly support her in building a new diet and managing her anxiety, the most important thing was that she put herself in a position to help herself. If her emotional eating continued, there was no way her antianxiety diet would be effective.

My discussion with Kayu was inspired by a philosophy called intuitive eating. While dieting can show results for weight loss and general health in the short term, studies have shown that food restriction has limited success over the long term. In fact, there is evidence that dieting not only leads to an increased risk of further weight gain five years later[22] but also encourages your brain to associate food with reward and attention.[23] Intuitive eating was first developed in 1995 by nutritionists Evelyn Tribole and Elyse Resch, who sought an alternative to this unhealthy and ineffective diet culture.

The central idea of intuitive eating is that rather than limiting your diet to certain types or amounts of food, you take cues from your body to determine what and how much you should eat. As we saw with the Blue Zones' 80 Percent Rule, you focus on letting your body tell you when you are full, rather than eating habitually or reactively, overstuffing yourself just because food is available or because it makes you feel good in the moment. Intuitive eating and the ten principles that underpin it have been written about extensively in other books, so I won't go into a great deal of detail here, but I certainly encourage you to explore this thoughtful and helpful approach to eating.

Intuitive eating can be particularly challenging for people who suffer from anxiety; as with Kayu, anxiety can feel debilitating, keeping you from doing the things you know you need to do to help yourself. But developing an intuitive eating practice can also be particularly powerful for anxious people. As we've seen in many different cases in this book, anxiety can lead you to overeat or undereat,[24] distorting your feelings of hunger or fullness.[25] Add on the kinds of social pressures that Kayu was feeling to fit into her new culture and friend group, and it can be challenging to approach food in a mindful and measured way. But that also means there is great potential for reframing how you think about eating and developing a new relationship that will help calm your anxiety no matter what kind of diet you choose to follow.

To get Kayu started, I introduced her to a simple plan I've developed called Dr. Uma's Calm Diet. The idea is to help you understand that a diet is not meant to be a punitive tool. Diets are meant to provide frameworks for self-improvement based on your personal needs. Research demonstrates that shame, self-criticism, and perceptions of inferiority make you lose self-control and undermine the effectiveness of what you are trying to achieve by changing your eating habits.

Focus On:

- *Self-love and respect.* Knowing and honoring your needs is where self-love and respect begin. This is a pillar of helping yourself heal your anxiety.

- *Self-attunement.* Paying attention to body intelligence teaches you how to be in tune with your own body and brain, which can help you gauge the effects of different foods.

- *Self-listening.* Anxiety comes with different emotions for different people. Listening to your own triggers is key to helping you overcome your own specific brand of it.

- *Self-direction.* Being self-directed makes you feel empowered and in control of managing your anxiety by directing your self-love, self-attunement, and self-listening to lowering your anxiety.

- *Self-improvement.* As you work through the other steps, allow yourself to feel your improvement as you heal your anxiety.

Be Aware of:

- *Perfectionism.* Don't try to be perfect, especially when it comes to how you eat and feel. Everyone is going to make mistakes and have bad days. Have grace with yourself.

- *Criticism and judgment.* Stepping back from being harsh to yourself and others will help you release and lower anxiety.

- *Letting others lead you.* One of the positive impacts of nutritional psychiatry is that it gives you autonomy over the initial steps you can take to reducing your anxiety. While it's good to work with a trusted professional, don't let the popular press or social media lead you.

- *Self-hatred and criticism.* Practicing mindfulness and soothing self-hatred will help relieve anxiety triggers.

- *Putting your emotions before the whole you.* Your anxiety is a part of you, but you need to understand that it does not define you. By following the nutritional and integrative principles in this book, you can lessen the burden of anxiety on your whole self.

As I walked Kayu through these steps toward reframing her relationship with eating, I explained to her that I was not asking her to love her weight gain or her anxiety, but to give herself permission to listen to what she already knew. She did not believe that eating a plate of deep-fried tempura or chicken wings was good for her on a regular basis. Of course, these foods were delicious, but she cared about more than deliciousness. She cared about allowing her brain and body to feel their best. But she had lost sight of those priorities as she had understandably let her desire to fit in override everything else. Rather than self-criticizing, or letting her emotions convince her that there was no way to change, I encouraged her to get back in tune with how she ate in Japan.

She took in what I was saying and became more enthusiastic about finding ways to get back on track. Our plan was simple: We took an inventory of which Japanese foods agreed with the Six Pillars and looked for ways she could integrate them back into her diet. We discussed principles like hara hachi bu, which helped make her feel more culturally grounded in her eating. She told me she had never been much of a cook growing up, but I told her the same was true for me—I had relatives who were expert cooks; I never learned to cook many of the dishes I grew up eating until I was studying later and living on my own. She made a point to ask her own relatives for recipes and cooking tips, as well as enrolling in a Japanese cooking class that was offered nearby. As she began to cook for herself more, she prioritized healthier options like sushi, steamed vegetables, and fresh salads, avoiding tempura and fast food.

With these changes—and without using any medication, which she wanted to avoid at all costs—Kayu was able to go back to cutting hair with a steady hand. In six months, she lost twenty pounds and became the version of herself she wanted to be.

THE BEST DIET IS THE ONE THAT WORKS FOR YOU

My years of clinical work have reinforced time and again that every person eats differently. All of us have different cultural backgrounds, different palates, different food priorities. Every one of our bodies and gut microbiomes reacts to food in different ways. It would be foolish to try to fit every single person into a single dietary template. In fact, I suspect this is a major reason diets don't work for most people. How we eat is how we live, it's not separate, so aligning our true values with the foods we eat is crucial to live our best lives.

Apart from the foods we choose to eat, some people hate to follow a regimented eating schedule with each meal planned weeks in advance. Others absolutely love the structure and knowing in advance what they are going to eat. Some have more self-control over their food choices than others. Some cook by feel, adding a pinch of this and a dash of that. Others enjoy getting out the food scale to weigh out portions down to the gram.

In this chapter, I hope I've impressed upon you that different ways of eating are perfectly fine, as long as you are following the Six Pillars to Calm Your Mind. By combining those principles with the basics of the best diets out there, and listening to your body through intuitive eating, you have the power to construct a revolutionary personalized plan to control *your* anxiety with food.

CHAPTER THIRTEEN

Cooking Tips for a Calm Kitchen

Finally, we finish our quest to calm our minds with food in my favorite place: the kitchen. Kitchens have always been a place of comfort and calm to me, from my days as a child when my multi-generational family cooked healthy and mouthwatering food to enjoy together, to my time in medical school, when my love for Julia Child led to my devouring every episode of *The French Chef* on PBS. Now one of the greatest joys I experience as a nutritional psychiatrist is seeing my patients who don't have a strong connection with cooking learn to love the kitchen as much as I do, coming to see it as a place where they can both nourish their body and calm their mind.

If you're intimidated by the prospect of cooking meals from scratch rather than heating up prepared meals, here are some tips for cooking equipment and techniques.

What basic equipment should every cook have in their kitchen?

I must confess I love everything in the kitchen, from the food itself to each tool and utensil I use. It's my playground and my canvas, and it brings me joy and a sense of calm. It's my happy place.

I only began cooking later in life. When I was growing up, in a multigenerational South Asian family, my beloved late grand-mother, aunts, older cousins, and mom always took care of the meals. Of course, I assisted in the kitchen, learning to shell fresh peas or picking stones and debris out of trays of dried lentils before they were cooked. But since I was never in charge of the main parts of the meal, when I began cooking, I learned to assess what worked best for me through trial and error. After figuring some things out on my own, I went to culinary school to refine my knowledge, adding classical cooking training to my skills.

While peeking into a kitchen store is enough to let you know that there is an almost unlimited range of kitchen tools and gadgets, the fundamental tools are fairly simple. Here is a list of the basics you'll need, along with a few specialized favorites.

- *A pot and a pan, with lids, along with a rimmed sheet pan.* A good-quality 4–6-quart pot, a 10-inch frying pan, and a cast-iron skillet will be the workhorses of your kitchen. In the pot, you can simmer or boil lentils, beans, and legumes; make soups and curries; and steam your favorite veggies. The frying pan is for cooking eggs, a tofu scramble, or a colorful, fiber-rich stir-fry. The sheet pan is perfect for baking salmon or roasting vegetables.

- *A chef's knife.* Find a knife you are comfortable with. Most trained chefs are taught to use an 8- or 10-inch chef's knife for all tasks (I prefer an 8-inch knife), but using a large knife to cut small ingredients takes practice, and many home cooks prefer to have a range of smaller paring knives. Either way, keep your knife sharpened, as blunt knives can more easily slip and lead to dangerous cuts. As long as you can keep them sharp, there's nothing wrong with using less expensive knives as you develop your own preferences for the style or size, and then you can go for a higher-quality blade that will last a lifetime.

- A *vegetable peeler.* Having a peeler on hand is key. If you compost, save those peels for your garden or local composting site. While I prefer to peel certain vegetables and fruits—like carrots and mangoes—always leave the peels on if the recipe gives you the option, as they carry a high concentration of fiber and polyphenols.

- A *zester.* Citrus is an amazing natural, delicious flavor booster and is rich in antioxidants. Adding lemon, lime, or orange zest to a salad, soup, smoothie, or even tea is an inexpensive, brain-healthy way to amp up flavor. Keep sliced citrus for your water bottle, too. If you juice a lemon or lime but don't use all of the peel, you can always freeze the peel to zest later.

- A *cutting board.* I love a high-quality wood cutting board, but there are also great sustainable options made from recycled and repurposed materials. While I don't mind a cheap knife to start you off, I don't recommend a cheap plastic cutting board. Spending a bit more on a wooden board, or a BPA-free synthetic board, is best, as toxins can leach into your food from a cheap plastic board. One of the things drilled into us in culinary school was good food-safety practices. If you prepare meat and seafood, you should always wash your board with detergent and hot water after using it, and you should flip it over before you chop another food to avoid cross contamination.

- A *bench scraper.* During my early days studying at the Culinary Institute of America, I was introduced to an unfamiliar tool that became one of my kitchen all-stars. A bench scraper is a simple sheet of stiff metal with a handle on one side. Though it's traditionally used by bakers when making dough, a bench scraper can be used to scoop up chopped veggies or anything else from your cutting board, making it easy to transfer them to a pot or salad bowl.

- *A set of smaller stainless-steel or glass bowls for meal prep and mise en place, and larger bowls for serving food.* "Mise en place" is a phrase from French cuisine that means "everything in its place." This is one of the most important concepts I learned in culinary school. Before you start combining ingredients in a dish, take the time to wash, chop, and prep each ingredient and place it in its own small bowl. Then, once the heat is on, everything is ready at your fingertips, leaving you free to make sure you're cooking things properly.

- *Sustainable dishwashing sponges and a good-quality dish soap.* I buy sustainable sponges, which I wash in soap and hot water every night and allow to air dry. I recycle these regularly.

Are there any easy techniques you learned in your culinary training that you think every home cook should know?

- Get comfortable experimenting with different spices and spice blends to make your food both flavorful and healthy. It's an unfortunate myth that healthy food can't be delicious, and basic spices can really liven up a meal and provide anxiety-busting benefits.

- Learn to blanch and shock vegetables so you retain their flavor and nutrient value. For instance, if I were cooking purple sprouting broccoli, I would give it a quick 3–4-minute immersion in boiling salted water and then plunge it into an ice bath. This process stops the cooking instantly so the vegetable retains its color and nutrients and doesn't become soggy.

- Peel ginger with the back of a spoon; a knife or peeler is often not suitable for ginger's irregular, knobby shape. Peeled ginger can be frozen for later use. The clean peels can be steeped into a flavorful tea.

- If you need to cut dark chocolate, use a serrated knife. It will chop more easily, and the knife is much less likely to slip.

CHAPTER FOURTEEN

Recipes to Calm Your Mind

BREAKFAST

Basil Seed Pudding

Vegetarian, gluten-free, dairy-free

In my childhood we drank a sugar-laden milkshake called falooda, which contained ice cream, rose syrup, and a layer of basil seeds floating on top. Though true falooda is far too sweet to be brain-healthy, it inspired me to create this healthy pudding and my own version of bubble tea (see page 268), which tap into the antianxiety powers of basil seeds. Like chia and flaxseeds, basil seeds are rich in fiber, protein, and micro-nutrients, promoting good gut health. When soaked in liquid, they create a pudding that makes a great, satisfying breakfast. I like to top mine with hazelnuts and blueberries.

Servings: 1
Prep Time: 10 minutes; setting time 1–6 hours or overnight

2 tablespoons basil seeds

$^3/_4$ cup hemp milk (or milk of choice)

$^1/_2$ teaspoon manuka honey

$^1/_2$ teaspoon vanilla extract

$^1/_4$ teaspoon ground cardamom

$^1/_4$ cup blueberries

Whisk together all the ingredients except the blueberries in a 16-ounce measuring cup or medium glass bowl. Pour into a 4-ounce ramekin. Cover and allow to set overnight in the refrigerator. The next morning the bottom of the pudding may be thick and the top more liquid. If so, stir the pudding thoroughly, and the thickness should even out. This recipe is not sweet, so add some blueberries as a topping to sweeten it up naturally.

Chef's Tips:

- Pudding(s) will last about 5 days in the fridge sealed with plastic wrap, so you can do breakfast meal prep for the week ahead.
- A 4-ounce ramekin is the right size for breakfast, but you can also split the pudding into 2 (2-ounce) ramekins to eat as a snack.
- Add chocolate flavor by warming the milk and mixing in 1 teaspoon dark cacao powder. Allow to cool before adding in basil seeds and other ingredients.

Chickpea Scramble

Vegan, gluten-free

This no-egg scramble is a terrific way to start your day with the power of legumes, vegetables, and spices. It also makes a satisfying lunch or dinner when paired with a salad or vegetable side.

Servings: 1
Prep Time: 10 minutes
Cooking Time: 10 minutes

- 1/4 cup chickpea flour
- 1/4 teaspoon kosher salt
- 1/4 teaspoon black pepper
- 1/2 teaspoon ground turmeric
- 1/2 teaspoon garlic powder
- 1/2 teaspoon onion powder
- 1/4 teaspoon cayenne pepper
- Pinch of garam masala
- 1/4 cup nutritional yeast
- 1 tablespoon avocado oil or clarified butter
- 1 scallion, sliced
- 1/4 cup sliced mushrooms
- 1/4 cup baby spinach
- 1 tablespoon chopped fresh cilantro

Mix the flour, salt, spices, and nutritional yeast in a medium bowl. Add 1/3 cup water and whisk into a batter.

Heat the oil in a 10-inch pan. Add the scallion, mushrooms, and spinach and sauté until softened, about 5 minutes.

Pour in the batter and cook on medium heat until the scramble is cooked. Move the mixture around the pan with a spatula as you would do for scrambled eggs, for about 5 minutes.

Garnish with chopped cilantro.

Brain-Food Granola

Vegetarian, gluten-free

Packaged granola tends to be high in added sugars and processed ingredients, but it's very easy to make your own healthy, delicious granola at home. My version is packed with nuts, seeds, and spices, and it's great served with yogurt or eaten alone as a snack. I like to make a big batch, which lasts about a month stored in a sealed glass jar.

Servings: 20
Prep Time: 10 minutes
Cooking Time: 1 hour

- 2 tablespoons coconut oil
- 3 tablespoons raw honey or manuka honey
- 2 tablespoons ground cinnamon
- 1 tablespoon ground ginger
- 1 teaspoon ground nutmeg
- 1 cup crushed walnuts
- 1 cup crushed almonds
- 2½ cups rolled oats
- 2 tablespoons flaxseeds
- 2 tablespoons hemp seeds
- 1 cup sunflower seeds
- 1 cup pumpkin seeds

Preheat the oven to 300°F. Line a sheet pan with parchment paper.

Heat the oil in a medium pot over low heat. Add the honey and spices.

In a large bowl, mix the nuts, oats, and seeds. Pour in the oil, honey, and spice mix. Mix thoroughly and spread out on the sheet pan.

Roast for 1 hour, until golden brown, stirring the granola mix every 15 minutes to prevent it from burning. Cool and serve.

Quinoa Cereal

Vegetarian, gluten-free

This hearty, comforting breakfast is a healthy twist on the classic bowl of oatmeal. Though quinoa cereals are becoming more common in stores, making it from scratch ensures you avoid the processed ingredients often present in store-bought versions. Quinoa is rich in protein, fiber, and a variety of micronutrients. I like to top it with blueberries, 1 tablespoon unsweetened coconut flakes, or 1 ounce extra-dark chocolate chunks.

Servings: 2
Prep Time: 15 minutes
Cooking Time: 10 minutes

  ½ cup quinoa

  1½ cups hemp milk (or milk of choice)

  2 teaspoons applesauce

  1 teaspoon manuka (or other) honey

  ¼ teaspoon ground cinnamon

  Pinch of grated nutmeg

Rinse the quinoa using a strainer. Bring the milk and quinoa to a boil in a small saucepan. Reduce the heat to low and simmer, covered, until most of the milk is absorbed, about 10 minutes.

Remove from the heat and stir in the applesauce, honey, and cinnamon. Sprinkle with grated nutmeg.

Chef's Tip:

- For added creamy deliciousness and anxiety-beating omegas, add a tablespoon of seed-and-nut butter as an option.

LUNCH AND DINNER
Burmese Chickpea Tofu

Vegan, gluten-free

This chickpea-based tofu makes for a delicious alternative to familiar soy tofu, offering a bit of variety that's also packed with fiber and nutrients. Once prepared, it can be cut into small chunks and used in any recipe that calls for tofu.

Servings: 5
Prep Time: 10 minutes
Cooking Time: 15 minutes plus 2 hours to set

1 cup chickpea flour

1/2 teaspoon kosher salt

1/4 teaspoon ground turmeric

1 teaspoon garlic powder

1 teaspoon onion powder

1/2 teaspoon paprika

Pinch of black pepper

Line a lidded 8-by-8-inch glass dish with parchment paper.

Boil 1½ cups water in a medium saucepan.

In a medium glass bowl, whisk all the ingredients with 1 cup cold water until the mixture is smooth.

Lower the heat to medium, then slowly pour the chickpea mixture into the boiling water, whisking gently to combine.

Allow to cook for about 4 minutes on low to medium heat, then pour the thickened mixture into the glass dish, using a spatula to gently spread it out into a smooth layer. Some of the mixture may stick to the bottom of the pan and that is to be expected. Remove as much as you can.

Cover the glass dish with the lid and place in the fridge to cool. Allow to chill for 2 hours. Drain off any remaining liquid, and cut and use as desired.

Crispy Tikka Masala Tofu

Vegan, gluten-free

There are a multitude of ways to prepare tofu, but my favorite is to get it nice and crispy in an air fryer. This version includes South Asian spices, but it's adaptable to many other flavor profiles by altering the spice blend used. Bump up the spices if you like foods more spicy. And add this to my Go-To Calm Green Salad on page 255 as your protein.

Servings: 4
Prep Time: 10 minutes
Cooking Time: 20 minutes

2 tablespoons avocado oil

1 teaspoon red chili powder

½ teaspoon garam masala

1 teaspoon ground turmeric

¼ teaspoon black pepper

½ teaspoon ground coriander

½ teaspoon ground cumin

½ teaspoon onion powder

½ teaspoon garlic powder

1 teaspoon kosher salt

8-ounce block firm organic non-GMO tofu, or 8 ounces Burmese Chickpea Tofu (238)

Mix the avocado oil, spices, and salt in a large bowl.

Drain the tofu. Place in a medium baking dish and cover with parchment paper. Place a sheet pan on top of the parchment paper and weigh the pan down with 2 heavy tins of canned food. Press the tofu for 30 minutes. Uncover and drain the excess liquid.

Cut the block of tofu into ½- to 1-inch cubes. After placing the pieces in your air fryer pan/basket, sprinkle on the oil-spice mixture.

Bake in an air fryer at 375°F for 10–12 minutes or until golden and crispy (about 8 minutes if you prefer a softer texture), or bake in an oven set to 375°F for 15–20 minutes, depending on how soft or crisp you prefer.

Healthy-ish Mac and Cheese

Vegetarian

Mac and cheese is a comfort food for many, but most versions are quite unhealthy. My version of this classic replaces most of the cheese with a cauliflower puree for cruciferous goodness. Cooking the pasta ahead and cooling it fully before combining it into the dish helps reduce its glycemic index. Adjust the nutritional yeast and replace the Parmesan and cheddar with a vegan option to make this recipe vegan.

Servings: 6
Prep Time: 20 minutes
Cooking Time: 15 minutes

1½ cups macaroni

2 cups frozen cauliflower florets

1½ cups almond milk (or milk of choice)

1 teaspoon kosher salt

¼ teaspoon black pepper

2 tablespoons nutritional yeast

1 clove garlic, chopped

1 teaspoon chopped fresh parsley

1 teaspoon chopped fresh thyme

¼ cup grated Parmesan cheese

1 tablespoon olive oil

½ cup grated cheddar cheese

For the Pasta:

At least an hour before making the dish, boil salted water in a medium pot and cook the macaroni per the instructions on the box. This will yield roughly 3 cups cooked macaroni. Drain and cool in the fridge. Macaroni can be stored in an airtight container in the fridge for up to 3 days.

For the Mac and Cheese:

Preheat the oven to 375°F.

Place the cauliflower in a medium glass bowl and steam in the microwave for 2–3 minutes, or until soft and tender.

Add the cauliflower and milk to a food processor or blender and blend until smooth (if it's too thick, like a paste, add more milk until it has the consistency of a sauce).

Pour the mixture into a medium saucepan and bring to a simmer over low heat. Add the salt, pepper, nutritional yeast, garlic, and herbs, stirring gently. Simmer for 5 minutes.

Add the cooled macaroni to the warm sauce. Gently mix in the Parmesan cheese and olive oil. Pour the mixture into a 9-by-9-inch square baking dish. Sprinkle with the cheddar cheese.

Bake for 10–15 minutes or until the top is golden and bubbling.

Chef's Tips:

- Top with crushed almonds for crunch and texture.
- For added protein, sauté organic grass-fed ground sirloin or ground turkey with onions, salt, and pepper and add this to your sauce.
- If using dried parsley or thyme, just halve the amount, as dried herbs are more concentrated.

Korean-Indian Baked Chicken

Gluten-free

Baked chicken is a healthy and easy-to-prepare protein option, and it makes for a great meal with vegetable sides. This recipe uses both gochugaru, a Korean chili powder, and Kashmiri chili powder for heat and flavor. Good-quality organic versions of these spices can be found at an ethnic supermarket or online. If you have trouble finding either one, they can be replaced with cayenne pepper or paprika.

Servings: 2
Prep Time: 5 minutes plus at least 30 minutes for marinating
Cooking Time: 30 minutes

- ½ teaspoon Kashmiri chili powder
- ½ teaspoon gochugaru
- 1 teaspoon ground turmeric
- ¼ teaspoon black pepper
- ½ teaspoon ground coriander
- ½ teaspoon ground cumin
- ½ teaspoon garlic powder
- ½ teaspoon kosher salt
- 1 tablespoon avocado oil
- 2 (6-ounce) boneless, skinless chicken breasts
- 1 tablespoon chopped fresh cilantro

Mix the spices, salt, and oil in a large bowl. Combine the spice mixture with the chicken breasts and cover. Marinate in the refrigerator for at least 30 minutes, up to overnight.

When ready to cook, position a rack in the middle of the oven and preheat the oven to 400°F. Line a sheet pan with parchment paper.

Place the chicken breasts on the sheet pan and bake for about 30 minutes, or until the internal temperature at the thickest part of the breast reads 165–170°F. Garnish with cilantro.

Korean-Inspired Shrimp

Gluten-free

Shrimp is rich in protein, micronutrients (especially vitamin B_{12}), and brain-healthy omega-3 fatty acids. If you live in an area where fresh *seafood is readily available, fresh shrimp are best, but otherwise, frozen shrimp are widely available.*

Servings: 1
Prep Time: 10 minutes
Cooking Time: 3 minutes

> 8 medium shrimp, peeled and deveined, tails on
>
> 1 teaspoon gochugaru
>
> ½ teaspoon ground turmeric
>
> ¼ teaspoon black pepper
>
> ¼ teaspoon garlic powder
>
> ½ teaspoon kosher salt
>
> 1 tablespoon avocado oil

Toss the shrimp with the spices and salt.

Heat the oil in a cast-iron skillet over medium heat. Add the shrimp and stir-fry until they are cooked through and pink, about 3 minutes.

Masala Baked Salmon

Gluten-free

Fatty fish like salmon are the best source of omega-3s, and they're also a powerhouse for protein and micronutrients. Baked salmon is easy and flexible to prepare, and this recipe combines it with a South Asian masala made into a paste. If you prefer, the masala could also be used instead with oven-baked chicken or tofu.

Servings: 2
Prep Time: 10 minutes
Cooking Time: 8–12 minutes depending on internal temperature

2 (4–6-ounce) salmon fillets, deboned

2 tablespoons avocado oil

1 teaspoon Kashmiri chili powder

1 teaspoon ground turmeric

¼ teaspoon black pepper

½ teaspoon ground coriander

½ teaspoon ground cumin

½ teaspoon onion powder

½ teaspoon garlic powder

½ teaspoon kosher salt

1 tablespoon chopped fresh cilantro, optional

Preheat the oven to 350°F and line a baking sheet with parchment paper. Place the salmon on the baking sheet skin side down.

In a small glass bowl, whisk together the oil, spices, and salt to create a thick paste. Brush the salmon pieces with the masala paste. Bake for 8–12 minutes, or until the salmon is cooked through, to an internal temperature of 145°F. Garnish with cilantro, if desired.

Sambar (Dal)

Vegetarian, gluten-free

Dal, an Indian lentil stew, is one of my favorite brain-healthy comfort foods. Sambar is a version of dal popular in South India flavored with tamarind, a tropical fruit that produces pods containing a paste-like sweet-and-sour fruit. Tamarind concentrate is sold at specialty food stores and online. Read the label to make sure there are no added preservatives. Asafetida powder is used in Indian cooking as a digestive, helping to lower the effects of gas and bloating from foods like beans and lentils. While it has a pungent aroma, it is very flavorful once added to a dish.

Servings: 8
Prep Time: 30 minutes (plus overnight soaking)
Cooking Time: 30 minutes

- 2 cups yellow split pea lentils
- 2 tablespoons ghee or avocado oil
- 1 teaspoon black mustard seeds, optional
- 1 teaspoon cumin seeds
- 2 cloves garlic, peeled and sliced in half lengthwise
- 1 dried whole red chili, optional
- 1 medium onion, finely chopped
- 1 medium tomato, finely chopped
- 1 cup eggplant cut into 1-inch pieces
- 1 cup red pepper cut into 1-inch pieces
- 1 teaspoon ground turmeric
- 1/4 teaspoon black pepper
- 1 teaspoon tamarind paste concentrate
- 1 tablespoon kosher salt
- 1 teaspoon asafetida powder, optional
- 1 teaspoon chopped fresh cilantro

Rinse and soak the lentils in a covered glass bowl in the fridge overnight. Make sure the water covers the lentils by about 1/2 inch. Rinse the lentils the next day, transfer to a large saucepan, and add 4 cups water. Boil the lentils for about 30 minutes, until soft. The texture should be smooth, like a paste, so if necessary, you can smooth with an immersion blender. Alternatively, you can cook the lentils in a pressure cooker.

Heat the ghee in a medium stainless-steel pot over medium heat. Add the black mustard seeds, if using, and cook until they pop. Add the cumin seeds, garlic, red chili, if using, and chopped onion. Cook for 3–5 minutes, or until the onion is translucent. Add the tomato, eggplant, red pepper, turmeric, and black pepper, and stir to combine. Allow the mixture to sauté for 5 minutes, until tender.

Stir in the lentils, lower the heat, and add the tamarind paste and 2 cups water, stirring gently to combine. Allow to cook for about 20 minutes.

Season with the salt and the asafetida powder, if using. Serve hot, garnished with chopped cilantro.

Show-Stopping Roasted Head of Broccoli

Vegan, gluten-free

Broccoli is absolutely packed with all the nutritional benefits of cruciferous vegetables: low-glycemic-index carbs, fiber, micronutrients, and bioactives. This recipe is a great example of how vegetables can be the main course rather than just a side.

Servings: 4
Prep Time: 5 minutes
Cooking Time: 30 minutes

1 large head of broccoli

¼ cup avocado oil

1 tablespoon gochugaru

½ teaspoon ground turmeric

¼ teaspoon black pepper

1 teaspoon kosher salt

1 clove garlic, finely chopped

1 tablespoon chopped fresh cilantro

2 tablespoons lemon juice

1 tablespoon lemon zest

1 tablespoon pomegranate seeds

Preheat the oven to 425°F.

If the head of broccoli has a large stalk, cut it off at the base and sit the head firmly in a medium ovenproof baking dish.

Mix the oil with the spices, salt, garlic, and cilantro in a small bowl and pour the mixture over the head of broccoli.

Roast the broccoli in the oven for 20–25 minutes.

Top with fresh lemon juice, lemon zest, and pomegranate seeds before serving.

Chef's Tip:

• Save your broccoli stalks and chop them up for a soup or stir-fry.

Spaghetti Squash Noodles with Walnut "Pesto"

Vegan, gluten-free

Spaghetti squash is a terrific replacement for standard wheat pasta, providing noodle-y goodness without the blood sugar spike. In this recipe, our pesto leaves traditional Italian flavors behind for a MediterrAsian blend of fermented miso and spices combined with the healthy fats of walnuts. The rice wine vinegar offers a great umami flavor, but you can omit it if you don't have any on hand.

Servings: 4
Prep Time: 10 minutes
Cooking Time: 20 minutes

1 large spaghetti squash

2 tablespoons avocado oil

2 teaspoons kosher salt, divided

1 cup raw walnuts

¼ cup nutritional yeast

1 teaspoon gochugaru

½ teaspoon rice wine vinegar

1½ tablespoons white miso paste

1 teaspoon garlic powder

For the Squash:

Preheat the oven to 400°F. Line a sheet pan with parchment paper.

Cut the squash in half lengthwise and scoop out the seeds. Brush each half with oil, season with half the salt, and place facedown on the sheet pan.

Roast for 20–25 minutes, or until fork-tender. Allow the squash to cool and scoop out the "spaghetti" from the squash with a fork into a large bowl.

For the Pesto:

Blend the remaining ingredients in a food processor for 2–3 minutes, until the mixture is crumbly.

Add the pesto to the squash noodles and stir until well combined.

SALADS, SIDES, AND SOUPS
Baked (and Cooled) Potato

Vegetarian, gluten-free

While potatoes may be a few too many calories as an everyday food, I do love a baked potato either eaten plain as a side or with toppings as a full meal. This method of cooking and fully cooling helps lower the glycemic index of potatoes, making them healthier for your metabolism and gut.

Servings: 4
Prep Time: 3 minutes
Cooking Time: 45–60 minutes to bake plus 12 hours to cool

4 large russet baking potatoes

¼ cup avocado oil

1 tablespoon kosher salt

Preheat the oven to 450°F. Line a sheet pan with parchment paper.

Wash the potatoes thoroughly and pat dry with a clean towel. Using a fork, prick several holes in the skin of each potato. Gently rub oil onto each and sprinkle with salt.

Place the potatoes on the sheet pan and bake for 45–60 minutes, until each is fork-tender or your paring knife easily cuts into the surface.

Store the potatoes in the fridge, covered, overnight.

When ready to serve, warm the potatoes in the microwave for 2–3 minutes, or in an air fryer set to 350–375°F for 4 minutes. Serve the potatoes with your choice of toppings, such as butter, chives, Parmesan cheese, or Shiitake Bacon (see page 261). Use vegan options for butter or cheese as desired. Eat the skin for added fiber and nutrients.

Creamy Cannellini Bean and Greens Soup

Vegan, gluten-free

This soup combines the antianxiety powers of beans and leafy greens to create a delicious Mediterranean-style meal.

Servings: 6
Prep Time: 15 minutes
Cooking Time: 15 minutes

1 tablespoon avocado oil

$\frac{1}{2}$ cup chopped yellow onions

$1\frac{1}{2}$ teaspoons kosher salt

$\frac{1}{2}$ teaspoon white pepper

1 teaspoon garlic powder

$\frac{1}{2}$ teaspoon fresh thyme

2 cans organic cannellini beans, drained and rinsed

2 cups low-sodium vegetable stock

2 cups hemp milk, or plant-based milk of choice

2 cups baby spinach

Juice of $\frac{1}{2}$ lemon

1 tablespoon chopped fresh flat-leaf parsley

1 tablespoon toasted pepitas

Heat the oil in a large stainless-steel pot over medium heat. Sauté the onions with the salt, spices, and thyme for about 5 minutes, or until the onions are softened and golden. Add the beans and sauté for another 5 minutes.

Add the stock and milk and bring to a boil.

Remove from the heat and place the soup in a blender to liquefy, adding more stock if it is too thick. Another option is to just use an immersion blender to liquefy the soup while still in the pot, off the heat.

Add the spinach and lemon juice just before serving, allowing the greens to wilt into the soup.

Serve topped with chopped parsley and pepitas.

Curried Cauliflower and Coconut Soup

Vegan, gluten-free

This hearty soup capitalizes on the nutritional strength of cauliflower, as well as the brain-positive blend of turmeric and black pepper.

Servings: 8
Prep Time: 10 minutes
Cooking Time: 30 minutes

> 2 (16-ounce) bags frozen cauliflower florets
>
> 4 tablespoons avocado oil
>
> 1 yellow onion, diced
>
> 4 cloves garlic, chopped
>
> ½ teaspoon kosher salt
>
> ½ teaspoon ground turmeric
>
> 1 teaspoon cayenne
>
> ½ teaspoon nutmeg
>
> Pinch of black pepper
>
> 1 teaspoon gochujang
>
> 4 cups low-sodium vegetable stock
>
> 1 cup coconut milk
>
> Sprinkle of chopped almonds or pepitas, optional
>
> Chopped fresh cilantro

Preheat the oven to 425°F.

Place the cauliflower florets on a sheet pan and brush with 1 tablespoon of the oil. Roast for 20 minutes, until tender.

Heat the remaining oil in a large pot over medium heat. Once the oil is shimmering, add the onion and garlic. Cook, stirring occasionally, until the onion is translucent, 6–8 minutes.

Add the salt, spices, and roasted cauliflower to the pot. Pour in the stock and coconut milk. Bring the soup to a boil, then reduce the heat and simmer for about 15 minutes.

Let the soup cool slightly. Blend until smooth using a blender or an immersion blender.

Serve topped with almonds or pepitas, if desired, and chopped cilantro. For added fiber and nutrient density, top with crispy roasted broccoli florets.

Crispy MediterrAsian Okra Fries

Vegan, gluten-free

There is no denying that we all love French fries, even if they're unhealthy and can worsen anxiety. These okra fries are a much healthier way to scratch that itch, since okra is a good source of fiber and micronutrients.

Servings: 4
Prep Time: 20 minutes
Cooking Time: 20 minutes

1 pound okra

2 tablespoons avocado oil

1 tablespoon chickpea flour

1 tablespoon arrowroot powder

1½ teaspoons onion powder

1½ teaspoons garlic powder

1 teaspoon cumin

1 teaspoon ground coriander

1 teaspoon Kashmiri chili powder

½ teaspoon ground turmeric

¼ teaspoon black pepper

2 tablespoons chopped fresh cilantro, optional

Set the air fryer to 400°F, or preheat the oven to 425°F. Line the air fryer basket with a small piece of parchment paper.

Wipe the okra with a clean, damp kitchen towel and pat dry. Cut each okra down the center lengthwise. Place the okra on a sheet pan and drizzle with oil before tossing it with chickpea flour and arrowroot powder. Stir the spices together in a small bowl and sprinkle them over the okra.

Place the okra in the air fryer basket and cook for 10 minutes. Remove the basket, carefully flip the okra over, and cook for another 5–8 minutes, until crispy. You will get the best crunchy effect if you place the okra in a single layer and air fry in batches.

Or, if using an oven, place the okra in a single layer on a sheet pan lined with parchment paper, and bake for about 10 minutes or a few minutes longer so that they get crispy.

Top with chopped cilantro, if desired. Add a dairy or nondairy yogurt dip on the side, if desired.

Go-To Calm Green Salad

Vegan, gluten-free

Leafy greens are some of the most important foods in the fight against anxiety. There's nothing wrong with a simple side salad based on one type of green, but whenever I can, I like to combine several different greens into a huge, satisfying salad. This salad can be served on its own as a side, or with a protein to complete a meal.

Servings: 2
Prep Time: 15 minutes

1 cup baby arugula

1 cup chopped dandelion greens

1 cup chopped romaine lettuce

1 cup chopped baby bok choy

2 celery stalks, cut into ½-inch pieces

4 red, yellow, or orange bell peppers, sliced

½ English cucumber, diced

½ cup grape tomatoes, halved

2 tablespoons extra-virgin olive oil

2 tablespoons lemon zest

Juice of ½ lemon

½ teaspoon kosher salt

Pinch of black pepper

When you're ready to eat, toss all the ingredients in a large bowl and serve fresh. If you don't plan to serve the salad immediately, don't add the oil, lemon zest, or juice until you're ready to eat. You can store the salad in a covered glass or stainless-steel container for up to 4 days in the fridge. You can also serve with another of your favorite homemade vinaigrettes.

For a full meal, my favorite protein-rich toppings per serving are:

- ¼ medium avocado, sliced
- 2 tablespoons slivered almonds or chopped walnuts
- ½ cup broccoli sprouts
- ½ cup spicy chickpeas
- ½ cup air-fried spicy cubed tofu

Dr. Uma's Crunchy Kaleidoscope Salad

Vegan, gluten-free

As an alternative to a traditional leafy green salad, this beautiful multi-colored salad is filled with legumes and vegetables that are rich with antianxiety nutrients. If you like, top it with a protein source like hemp or chia seeds, or canned anchovies, oysters, or sardines.

Servings: 4
Prep Time: 20 minutes

For the Salad:

1 (15-ounce) can organic great northern beans, drained and rinsed

1 (15-ounce) can organic black beans, drained and rinsed

1 (10-ounce) bag frozen organic corn, thawed and drained

4 orange mini sweet bell peppers, diced

4 red mini sweet bell peppers, diced

4 yellow mini sweet bell peppers, diced

2 celery stalks, diced

4 Persian cucumbers, diced

1 small serrano pepper, finely chopped (remove seeds for
   less heat)

1/4 medium red onion, finely diced

1/2 cup fresh flat-leaf Italian parsley, finely chopped

1/2 cup fresh cilantro, finely chopped

1/4 cup fresh mint, finely chopped

1 tablespoon lime zest

For the Dressing:

1/2 cup extra-virgin olive oil

2 teaspoons honey

Juice of 1 1/2 limes

1 teaspoon kosher salt

1/2 teaspoon black pepper

To prepare the salad, mix all the ingredients in a large bowl. To
prepare the dressing, mix all the ingredients in a mason jar and
shake to emulsify. Toss the salad with the dressing.

MediterrAsian-Inspired Eggplant

Vegan, gluten-free

*Eggplant is common in Mediterranean and Asian cuisines, so it's a natu-
ral fit for a MediterrAsian side dish. Japanese eggplant is longer, thinner,
and a lighter purple than the more familiar Italian eggplant. (If you can't
find Japanese eggplant, you can substitute 1 large Italian eggplant, cut
into 1-inch-thick lengthwise slices, for this recipe). This dish is spicy!*

Servings: 4
Prep Time: 30 minutes
Cooking Time: 20 minutes

4 Japanese eggplants

2 tablespoons avocado oil

2 teaspoons sesame oil

1 tablespoon gochujang

2 teaspoons coconut aminos

1 teaspoon rice vinegar

½ teaspoon gochugaru

¼ teaspoon Kashmiri chili powder

¼ teaspoon ground cumin

¼ teaspoon ground coriander

2 scallions, finely chopped

1 tablespoon sesame seeds

1 small serrano pepper, finely chopped (remove seeds for less heat)

1 tablespoon chopped fresh cilantro

Preheat the oven to 400°F. Line a sheet pan with parchment paper.

Slice the eggplants in half lengthwise. Score the flesh side in a crisscross pattern. Brush this side with 1 tablespoon of the avocado oil.

Add the remaining 1 tablespoon avocado oil to a cast-iron skillet over medium heat. Sear the eggplants flesh side down for 3 minutes. Use tongs to transfer the eggplants onto the sheet pan, flesh side up.

Combine the sesame oil with the gochujang, coconut aminos, vinegar, and spices to make a sauce. Brush the eggplant with the sauce. Bake for 15 minutes, until the eggplants are golden in color. Sprinkle on the scallions, sesame seeds, chopped serrano pepper, and fresh cilantro before serving.

Miso-Infused Cipollini Onions and Green Beans

Vegan, gluten-free

Onions are a great source of prebiotic fiber, and green beans are full of micronutrients. I prefer the longer, skinnier variety of green beans, sometimes called French green beans or haricots verts, but any variety will do. I omitted salt, as miso is salty.

Servings: 4
Prep Time: 10 minutes
Cooking Time: 20–25 minutes

   ½ cup white miso paste

   2 tablespoons avocado oil

   2 cloves garlic, chopped

   ¼ teaspoon black pepper

   2 cups cipollini onions

   2 cups green beans, trimmed and sliced into 2-inch pieces

Preheat the oven to 425°F. Line a sheet pan with parchment paper.

Mix the miso paste, oil, garlic, and pepper in a large bowl. Toss in the cipollini onions and green beans and stir to combine.

Place the vegetables on the sheet pan, making sure they are arranged in a single layer. Roast in the oven for about 45 minutes, until the onions are caramelized and the green beans are tender. Since ovens vary, check the vegetables periodically, as they may be done a few minutes earlier or later. Frozen green beans will cook faster.

Pan-Seared Purple Sprouting Broccoli

Vegan, gluten-free

Purple sprouting broccoli is my favorite antianxiety superfood, which is why it is on the cover of this book. It delivers an even greater dose of helpful micronutrients and bioactives than regular green broccoli because of the anthocyanins that give it that glorious purple hue. If you can't find it at the grocery store, try a local farmers' market or even try growing it yourself.

Servings: 4
Prep Time: 5 minutes
Cooking Time: 15 minutes

>   1 pound purple sprouting broccoli
>
>   2 tablespoons avocado oil
>
>   2 cloves garlic, thinly sliced
>
>   1 teaspoon kosher salt
>
>   ½ teaspoon white pepper
>
>   ½ teaspoon dried parsley
>
>   1 teaspoon dried oregano
>
>   ½ lemon
>
>   Extra-virgin olive oil (optional)

Cut off the florets from the purple sprouting broccoli and slice the stems.

Heat the avocado oil in a cast-iron skillet over high heat. Add the garlic, salt, pepper, and herbs, and then add the broccoli. Sauté very quickly, tossing with a spatula for about 3 minutes.

Add a squeeze of lemon juice and a drizzle of extra-virgin olive oil, if desired, before serving.

Shiitake Bacon

Vegan, gluten-free

This plant-based version of bacon is a great treat to serve as a garnish for baked potatoes or salads, or even on its own as a side. Mushrooms contain powerful bioactives that help support a calm feeling. No added salt is needed, as the coconut aminos are salty enough.

Servings: 4
Prep Time: 10 minutes
Cooking Time: 15 minutes

- 1 teaspoon avocado oil
- 2 cups shiitake mushrooms, stemmed and sliced ¼-inch thick
- 1 tablespoon coconut aminos
- ¼ teaspoon black pepper
- ¼ teaspoon ground turmeric
- 1 teaspoon smoked paprika

Preheat the oven to 400°F.

Heat the oil in a cast-iron skillet over medium heat. Add the rest of the ingredients, stir to coat, and sauté for about 3 minutes.

Transfer the skillet to the oven and bake for 10 minutes, until the mushrooms are dry, brown, and crispy.

Spicy Crunchy Cucumber Salad

Vegan, gluten-free

This cool, fresh salad is a great accompaniment to almost any dish. My favorite cucumbers to use are Persian, which are smaller and narrower than standard or English cucumbers.

Servings: 4
Prep Time: 15 minutes

- 6 Persian cucumbers
- 1 teaspoon sesame oil
- 1 teaspoon avocado oil
- 2 tablespoons rice vinegar
- 1 tablespoon tamari
- 1 tablespoon coconut aminos
- $\frac{1}{2}$ teaspoon honey
- $\frac{1}{4}$ teaspoon kosher salt
- 3 cloves garlic, minced
- 1 teaspoon gochugaru
- 1 teaspoon sesame seeds

Slice the cucumbers into rounds, leaving the skin on. Place them in a small glass dish with a lid. Whisk the remaining ingredients in a small bowl. Pour the dressing over the cucumbers and toss.

Store, covered, in the fridge and serve chilled.

DESSERTS

Calm Chocolate Mousse

Vegan, gluten free

This plant-based chocolate mousse is a great way to get a chocolatey treat without the unhealthy ingredients that may be added in a store-bought mousse. It also has a dose of healthy fats from the avocado. Serve plain or with a pinch of pink Himalayan salt or red pepper flakes, a handful of unsalted pistachios, or a sprinkle of blood sugar–stabilizing cinnamon.

Servings: 1
Prep Time: 15 minutes

1 ripe banana

¼ large ripe avocado

3 tablespoons organic cacao powder

½ teaspoon manuka honey

Add all the ingredients to a food processor and blend until smooth.

Chill, covered, in the fridge until you are ready to serve. If desired, top with blueberries or strawberries and cacao nibs for an extra antioxidant boost.

Chocolate Hazelnut Spread

Vegan, gluten-free

I absolutely love Nutella, but it's packed with added sugar and unhealthy fats. This version hits the same flavor profile while being much healthier to eat with apple slices, celery sticks, or carrot sticks, or to add to a smoothie. This is a rich, decadent spread, so you need only a bit to be satisfied.

Servings: 12
Prep Time: 15 minutes
Cooking Time: 30 minutes

2½ cups peeled hazelnuts

²/₃ cup extra-dark chocolate

2 tablespoons coconut oil

1 tablespoon honey

1 tablespoon cacao powder

1 tablespoon vanilla extract

Preheat the oven to 350°F. Line a sheet pan with parchment paper.

Spread the hazelnuts out on the pan and bake for about 10 minutes, until lightly browned. Remove the nuts and let them cool for 30 minutes.

Meanwhile, melt the chocolate in a double boiler using the bain-marie method (see Chef's Tip). Keep the melted chocolate warm until the hazelnuts have cooled.

Place the cooled hazelnuts in a food processer and pulse until they are the texture of sand. Pour in the melted chocolate, coconut oil, honey, cacao powder, and vanilla extract. Pulse until smooth — this may need a strong food processor or a touch of hemp milk to help make the spread smooth and less chunky.

Pour the spread into a clean glass jar, seal tightly, and refrigerate for up to 3 months.

Chef's Tip:

• To melt chocolate in a double boiler (the bain-marie method), fill a stainless-steel saucepan one-third full of water. Put the chocolate in a heatproof glass bowl and place it over the saucepan so that its base does not touch the water. Heat the water over medium heat. Once the chocolate starts to melt, remove the bowl from the heat using an oven mitt, then gently stir the chocolate until fully melted.

Dark Chocolate Chili Truffles

Vegan, gluten-free

If you have an urge for chocolate candy but don't want to risk worsening your anxiety with added sugars, these truffles, naturally sweetened with bananas, can be a great choice. They are flavored with coffee and chili, but you could also flavor them with crushed nuts, unsweetened coconut, or any other options you enjoy.

Servings: 8
Prep Time: 20 minutes
Cooking Time: 30 minutes plus overnight to set

7 ounces extra-dark chocolate, grated

½ teaspoon decaffeinated espresso powder

2 ripe bananas

1 teaspoon chipotle chili powder

½ teaspoon Maldon sea salt

Line an 8-inch-square glass dish with a layer of plastic wrap covered by a layer of parchment paper. Chill the dish in the freezer for half an hour.

Melt the chocolate in a double boiler using the bain-marie method. Stir in the espresso powder.

Blend the bananas in a food processor until smooth. Combine the bananas with the melted chocolate, stirring gently.

Pour the mixture into the baking dish and use a spatula to smooth the surface. Sprinkle with chipotle powder and sea salt.

Place the dish in the freezer overnight to set.

Transfer the truffle mixture from the glass dish onto a clean chopping board, and slice into 1-inch squares for serving.

Store in the freezer for up to 1 month in a sealed container.

Dr. Uma's Cherry CALM Smoothie

Vegan, gluten-free

With a balance of low-glycemic-index carbohydrates, healthy fats, fiber, and protein, this chocolate and cherry protein smoothie makes for an excellent on-the-go breakfast that will keep you full and focused throughout your morning. If you like, you could add a tablespoon of chia, flax, or hemp seeds.

1 cup fresh or frozen cherries, pitted

1 scoop protein powder of choice

2 teaspoons unsweetened cacao powder

½ teaspoon cinnamon powder

1 tablespoon raw nut butter

1½ cups spinach

8 ounces hemp milk, or milk of choice

Blend all the ingredients in a blender until smooth.

BEVERAGES

Homemade Hemp Milk

Vegan, gluten-free

Hemp milk is my favorite milk alternative. It can be served as a drink or used in any recipes that call for milk. Use less water for a creamier, thicker milk. It's also easy to create flavored and lightly sweetened milks using dates for sweetness and various flavors.

Servings: 6
Prep Time: 5 minutes

½ cup hulled hemp seeds (hemp hearts)
Pinch of kosher salt

Add hemp seeds, salt, and 4 cups water to a blender. Blend for 1 minute or until the milk is creamy. Use clean cheesecloth or a nut-milk bag to strain the milk for a less grainy texture.

To store, pour the milk into a glass bottle and seal tightly. It will keep, refrigerated, for up to 5 days.

For Vanilla Milk:

Add ½ teaspoon vanilla extract and 1 pitted date softened in hot water to the mixture when blending.

For Chocolate Milk:

Add 2 tablespoons natural cacao powder and 1 pitted date softened in hot water to the mixture when blending.

For Strawberry Milk:

Add ½ cup fresh or frozen strawberries and 1 pitted date softened in hot water to the mixture when blending.

Matcha Green "Bubble" Tea

Vegan, gluten-free

Traditional bubble tea is delicious, but it's made with unhealthy sweetened fruit powders, sugar, and starchy tapioca pearls. Inspired by my childhood favorite, falooda, my version swaps tapioca pearls for brain-healthy soaked basil seeds and contains other calming ingredients.

Servings: 1
Prep Time: 40 minutes

- 1 teaspoon matcha
- ½ teaspoon cardamom powder
- ½ teaspoon basil seeds
- 1 cup almond or hemp milk
- 1 teaspoon honey
- ½ teaspoon vanilla extract
- ½ cup ice

Whisk the matcha and cardamom with ¼ cup boiling water and set aside to cool.

Place the basil seeds in 1 cup water. Allow them to soak and swell up for 30 minutes, then drain and rinse.

In a tall glass, add the cooled matcha tea and the milk, honey, and vanilla extract. Stir.

Add the basil seeds and ice. Serve with a straw.

Passionflower Tisane

Vegan, gluten-free

Passionflower is an herbal remedy that can ease anxiety. This simple recipe for herbal tea can be used with many different types of tea as well.

Servings: 1
Prep Time: 10 minutes

1 tablespoon dried passionflower

½ teaspoon honey (optional)

Place the passionflower in a medium teacup. Pour 1 cup of boiling water over the passionflower and steep for about 10 minutes. If you have a tea ball or other infuser, that will help too.

Strain the passionflower and sweeten the tea with the honey, if desired.

PLAYING YOUR WAY TO CALM
Lavender Play Dough

For this final, nonedible recipe, I want to share my favorite tactile way to tamp down anxiety. I love carrying a ball of this homemade play dough in my purse to squeeze when I'm feeling anxious or stressed. Instead of lavender, you may want to use other calming essential oils, like jasmine, lemon balm, organic sweet basil, or chamomile, to name a few. Even the process of making it is relaxing—kneading the dough is calming and fun.

Prep Time: 5 minutes
Cooking Time: 10 minutes

- 2 cups all-purpose flour
- ³/₄ cup kosher salt
- 4 teaspoons cream of tartar
- 1½ tablespoons coconut oil
- ½ tablespoon lavender essential oil
- Purple food coloring or food coloring of choice

Combine the flour, salt, and cream of tartar in a medium nonstick saucepan. Add 2 cups lukewarm water and the remaining ingredients, and stir continuously over medium heat until the dough has thickened and starts to form a ball, about 2 minutes.

When the ball is firm, remove from the heat. Transfer the ball to a clean bowl and allow to cool for 2 minutes. Knead the dough on the countertop until smooth, about 5 minutes.

Store in a clear BPA-free plastic bag for up to 2 months.

Acknowledgments

When I wrote my first book, *This is Your Brain on Food*, I had no idea that it would resonate so widely, and I feel so blessed that it has launched my work in mental health into the world more boldly than anything I could achieve within the confines of my clinic. My second book has been a journey to truly reaching those struggling with anxiety, a condition that inserts itself across every demographic. So I want to acknowledge every single patient, friend, family member, and colleague who shared their anxiety, which taught me so much and helped me develop the protocol of this book — that there is hope, that nutrition and the food we eat are the power at the end of our work.

To my oncology and surgical team: Dr. Eric Winer, Drs. Tari King, Adrienne Gropper Waks, Jennifer McKenna, NP, and all the staff at Dana-Farber (Boston) who helped me reach the survivorship landmark as I wrote this book.

My agents: Celeste, Sarah, Mia, Emily, and their entire team at PFLM who brought this book to life and rallied with me to make *This Is Your Brain on Food* a classic that is now backlisted.

My editor, Tracy: I feel blessed that she selected me, an unknown MD-author with a niche message in nutritional psychiatry — thanks for believing in my first book and for your ongoing encouragement.

Thanks to the entire team at Little Brown, Spark / Hachette: Jess, Jules, Karina, and the amazing foreign rights team. A very big thank-you to William — how fortunate I am to have worked closely with you another time.

To my mentors in science, medicine, psychiatry, and nutrition at Harvard and beyond: for standing by me and encouraging me every step of the way. People often find this an enigma, yet I've been fortunate to have all of you throughout my career.

To the Massachusetts General Psychiatry Academy: Dr. David Rubin, Jane Pimental, Shauna Futch, and the entire team: thank you for your enduring support in helping me bring forward the world's first academic course in nutritional and metabolic psychiatry at Harvard.

I was very honored to meet HRH the former Prince of Wales. He suggested we need clear guidance for the public on what healthy food is, and this led to the UK Food for Mood Campaign.

To Dr. Dixon, Amanda King, and the entire team at the UK College of Medicine: thank you for working with me to amplify the Food for Mood Campaign.

My team, who are true gems and who love this work as much as I do and work hard to share this with the world: Olivia, Andrea, Roshini, Connor, Vina, Tanusha, Sayuj and team, Angela Jill, and Alexis.

Finally, I could not have written this book without my besties, Srini, Rajiv, and Denise.

A big thank-you to my entire family: my late dad; my mum, who is still an absolute superstar at everything; my siblings, Vahini, Hesh, and Vishy. To my beloved late aunty Nimi, who passed away suddenly prior to this book being released: thank you for the cookbook you bought me and all that you taught me; I miss you terribly. To the rest of my lovely family: Kamil, Laura, Namitha, Nag, Sashen, and Sayuri. To Oisín, Orin, and Nyra, who are beautiful reminders that food is love, even when it's healthy food!

Notes

Chapter 1: Fighting the Global Anxiety Epidemic

1. APA Public Opinion Polls. American Psychiatric Association. Accessed February 15, 2023. https://psychiatry.org/news-room/apa-public-opinion-polls.
2. New Poll: COVID-19 Impacting Mental Well-Being: Americans Feeling Anxious, Especially for Loved Ones; Older Adults Are Less Anxious. American Psychiatric Association. March 25, 2020. Accessed February 15, 2023. https://psychiatry.org/News-room/News-Releases/new-poll-covid-19 -impacting-mental-well-being-amer.
3. After Two Years of COVID-19, Americans' Anxiety Turns to Global Events, Says APA Annual Mental Health Poll. American Psychiatric Association. May 22, 2022. Accessed February 15, 2023. https://psychiatry.org/news-room /news-releases/americans-anxiety-global-events.
4. As Midterms Approach, 79% of Americans Believe Mental Health Is a Public Health Emergency That Needs More Attention from Lawmakers. American Psychiatric Association. October 6, 2022. Accessed February 15, 2023. https://www.psychiatry.org/News-room/News-Releases/Midterms -poll-mental-health-priority.
5. Bandelow B, Michaelis S. Epidemiology of anxiety disorders in the 21st century. *Dialogues in Clinical Neuroscience.* 2015;17(3):327–35. https://doi.org /10.31887/dcns.2015.17.3/bbandelow.
6. Anxiety Disorders — Facts & Statistics. Anxiety & Depression Association of America. Accessed February 15, 2023. https://adaa.org/understanding -anxiety/facts-statistics.
7. McLean CP, Asnaani A, Litz BT, Hofmann SG. Gender differences in anxiety disorders: Prevalence, course of illness, comorbidity and burden of illness. *Journal of Psychiatric Research.* 2011;45(8):1027–35. https://doi .org/10.1016/j.jpsychires.2011.03.006.

8. Eken HN, Dee EC, Powers AR III, Jordan A. Racial and ethnic differences in perception of provider cultural competence among patients with depression and anxiety symptoms: A retrospective, population-based, cross-sectional analysis. *Lancet Psychiatry.* 2021;8(11):957–68. https://doi.org /10.1016/s2215-0366(21)00285-6.

9. HHS Leaders Urge States to Maximize Efforts to Support Children's Mental Health. May 25, 2022. Accessed February 15, 2023. https://www.hhs.gov /about/news/2022/05/25/hhs-leaders-urge-states-maximize-efforts-support -childrens-mental-health.html.

10. Baumgaertner E. Health panel recommends anxiety screening for all adults under 65. *New York Times.* September 20, 2022. Accessed February 15, 2023. https://www.nytimes.com/2022/09/20/health/anxiety-screening -recommendation.html.

11. Karlsen HR, Matejschek F, Saksvik-Lehouillier I, Langvik E. Anxiety as a risk factor for cardiovascular disease independent of depression: A narrative review of current status and conflicting findings. *Health Psychology Open.* 2021;8(1):205510292098746. https://doi.org/10.1177/2055102920987462.

12. Chien IC, Lin CH. Increased risk of diabetes in patients with anxiety disorders: A population-based study. *Journal of Psychosomatic Research.* 2016;86:47–52. https://doi.org/10.1016/j.jpsychores.2016.05.003.

13. Siegmann EM, Müller HHO, Luecke C, Philipsen A, Kornhuber J, Grömer TW. Association of depression and anxiety disorders with autoimmune thyroiditis. *JAMA Psychiatry.* 2018;75(6):577. https://doi.org/10.1001 /jamapsychiatry.2018.0190.

14. Becker E, Orellana Rios CL, Lahmann C, Rücker G, Bauer J, Boeker M. Anxiety as a risk factor of Alzheimer's disease and vascular dementia. *British Journal of Psychiatry.* 2018;213(5):654–60. https://doi.org/10.1192/bjp.2018.173.

15. Murniati N, Al Aufa B, Kusuma D, Kamso S. A scoping review on biopsychosocial predictors of mental health among older adults. *International Journal of Environmental Research and Public Health.* 2022;19(17):10909. https://doi.org/10.3390/ijerph191710909.

16. Yaribeygi H, Panahi Y, Sahraei H, Johnston TP, Sahebkar A. The impact of stress on body function: A review. *EXCLI Journal.* 2017;16:1057–72. https:// doi.org/10.17179/excli2017-480. PMID: 28900385; PMCID: PMC5579396.

17. Barrett, LF. The theory of constructed emotion: An active inference account of interoception and categorization. *Social Cognitive and Affective Neuroscience.* 2017;12(1):1–23. https://doi.org/10.1093/scan/nsw154.

18. McRae K, Hughes B, Chopra S, Gabrieli JDE, Gross JJ, Ochsner KN. The neural bases of distraction and reappraisal. *Journal of Cognitive*

Neuroscience. 2010;22(2):248–62. https://doi.org/10.1162/jocn.2009.21243; Ellard KK, Barlow DH, Whitfield-Gabrieli S, Gabrieli JDE, Deckersbach T. Neural correlates of emotion acceptance vs worry or suppression in generalized anxiety disorder. *Social Cognitive and Affective Neuroscience.* 2017;12(6):1009–21. https://doi.org/10.1093/scan/nsx025; Taren AA, Gianaros PJ, Greco CM, et al. Mindfulness meditation training alters stress-related amygdala resting state functional connectivity: A randomized controlled trial. *Social Cognitive and Affective Neuroscience.* 2015;10(12):1758–68. https://doi.org/10.1093/scan/nsv066.

19. Barrett LF. You Aren't at the Mercy of Your Emotions. Presented at TED@ IBM; filmed December 2017 in San Francisco, CA. TED video, 18:20. Accessed July 11, 2022. https://www.ted.com/talks/lisa_feldman_barrett _you_aren_t_at_the_mercy_of_your_emotions_your_brain_creates_them ?language=en.

20. Mobbs D, Adolphs R, Fanselow MS, et al. Viewpoints: Approaches to defining and investigating fear. *Nature Neuroscience.* 2019;22(8):1205–16. https://doi.org/10.1038/s41593-019-0456-6.

21. Tiller JW. Depression and anxiety. *Medical Journal of Australia.* 2013;199(S6):S28–S31. https://doi.org/10.5694/mja12.10628.

22. Collier S. What Should You Do During a Psychiatric Medication Shortage? *Harvard Health Blog.* July 2, 2020. Accessed February 15, 2023. https://www .health.harvard.edu/blog/what-should-you-do-during-a-psychiatric -medication-shortage-2020070220526.

23. Kaczkurkin AN, Foa EB. Cognitive-behavioral therapy for anxiety disorders: An update on the empirical evidence. *Dialogues in Clinical Neuroscience.* 2015;17(3):337–46. https://doi.org/10.31887/dcns.2015.17.3/akaczkurkin.

24. Weiner S. A Growing Psychiatrist Shortage and an Enormous Demand for Mental Health Services. Association of American Medical Colleges. August 9, 2022. Accessed February 17, 2023. https://www.aamc.org/news -insights/growing-psychiatrist-shortage-enormous-demand-mental-health -services.

25. Bulkes NZ, Davis K, Kay B, Riemann BC. Comparing efficacy of telehealth to in-person mental health care in intensive-treatment-seeking adults. *Journal of Psychiatric Research.* 2022;145:347–52. https://doi.org/10.1016 /j.jpsychires.2021.11.003.

26. Orme-Johnson DW, Barnes VA. Effects of the Transcendental Meditation technique on trait anxiety: A meta-analysis of randomized controlled trials. *Journal of Alternative and Complementary Medicine.* 2014;20(5):330–41. https://doi.org/10.1089/acm.2013.0204.

27. Novaes MM, Palhano-Fontes F, Onias H, et al. Effects of yoga respiratory practice (bhastrika pranayama) on anxiety, affect, and brain functional connectivity and activity: A randomized controlled trial. *Frontiers in Psychiatry*. 2020;11. https://doi.org/10.3389/fpsyt.2020.00467.

28. Kandola A, Stubbs B. Exercise and anxiety. *Advances in Experimental Medicine and Biology*. 2020;1228:345–52. https://doi.org/10.1007/978-981-15 -1792-1_23.

29. Haghighatdoost F, Feizi A, Esmaillzadeh A, et al. Drinking plain water is associated with decreased risk of depression and anxiety in adults: Results from a large cross-sectional study. *World Journal of Psychiatry*. 2018;8(3):88– 96. https://doi.org/10.5498/wjp.v8.i3.88.

30. One in Four Americans Plans a Mental Health New Year's Resolution for 2022. American Psychiatric Association. December 20, 2021. Accessed February 15, 2023. https://psychiatry.org/News-room/News-Releases/One-in -Four-Americans-Plans-a-Mental-Health-New-Ye.

31. Roy-Byrne P. Treatment-refractory anxiety; definition, risk factors, and treatment challenges. *Dialogues in Clinical Neuroscience*. 2015;17(2): 191–206.

32. World Obesity Day 2022—Accelerating Action to Stop Obesity. World Health Organization. March 4, 2022. Accessed February 15, 2023. https:// www.who.int/news/item/04-03-2022-world-obesity-day-2022-accelerating -action-to-stop-obesity.

33. Adult Obesity Facts. Centers for Disease Control and Prevention. Accessed February 15, 2023. https://www.cdc.gov/obesity/data/adult.html.

Chapter 2: Gut Feelings

1. Lichtenstein GR. Letter from the editor. *Gastroenterology and Hepatology*. 2013 Sep;9(9):552. PMID: 24729764; PMCID: PMC3983972.

2. Pariente N. A Field Is Born. *Nature Portfolio*. June 17, 2019. Accessed February 15, 2023. https://www.nature.com/articles/d42859-019-00006-2.

3. Mackowiak PA. Recycling Metchnikoff: Probiotics, the intestinal microbiome and the quest for long life. *Frontiers in Public Health*. 2013;1. https:// doi.org/10.3389/fpubh.2013.00052.

4. Lederberg J, McCray AT. Ome SweetOmics—a genealogical treasury of words. *Scientist*. 2001;15(7):8.

5. Jefferson T. Thomas Jefferson to Maria Cosway, October 12, 1786. Founders Online. Accessed February 15, 2023. https://founders.archives.gov/documents /Jefferson/01-10-02-0309.

6. Yu CD, Xu QJ, Chang RB. Vagal sensory neurons and gut-brain signaling. *Current Opinion in Neurobiology.* 2020;62:133–40. https://doi.org/10.1016/j .conb.2020.03.006.

7. North CS. Relationship of functional gastrointestinal disorders and psychiatric disorders: Implications for treatment. *World Journal of Gastroenterology.* 2007;13(14):2020. https://doi.org/10.3748/wjg.v13.i14.2020.

8. Mohammad S, Chandio B, Soomro AA, et al. Depression and anxiety in patients with gastroesophageal reflux disorder with and without chest pain. *Cureus.* Published online November 8, 2019. https://doi.org/10.7759 /cureus.6103.

9. Goodwin RD. Generalized anxiety disorder and peptic ulcer disease among adults in the United States. *Psychosomatic Medicine.* 2002;64(6):862–66. https://doi.org/10.1097/01.psy.0000038935.67401.f3.

10. Bull MJ, Plummer NT. Part 1: The human gut microbiome in health and disease. *Integrative Medicine (Encinitas, Calif.).* 2014;13(6):17–22.

11. Martino C, Dilmore AH, Burcham ZM, Metcalf JL, Jeste D, Knight R. Microbiota succession throughout life from the cradle to the grave. *Nature Reviews Microbiology.* Published online July 29, 2022. https://doi.org/10.1038 /s41579-022-00768-z.

12. Human Microbiome Project. National Institutes of Health. Accessed February 15, 2023. https://commonfund.nih.gov/hmp.

13. Vijay A, Valdes AM. Role of the gut microbiome in chronic diseases: A narrative review. *European Journal of Clinical Nutrition.* 2021;76(4):489–501. https://doi.org/10.1038/s41430-021-00991-6; Durack J, Lynch SV. The gut microbiome: Relationships with disease and opportunities for therapy. *Journal of Experimental Medicine.* 2018;216(1):20–40. https://doi.org/10.1084 /jem.20180448.

14. Ursell LK, Metcalf JL, Parfrey LW, Knight R. Defining the human microbiome. *Nutrition Reviews.* 2012;70:S38–S44. https://doi.org/10.1111/j.1753 -4887.2012.00493.x.

15. Smits SA, Leach J, Sonnenburg ED, et al. Seasonal cycling in the gut microbiome of the Hadza hunter-gatherers of Tanzania. *Science.* 2017;357(6353): 802–6. https://doi.org/10.1126/science.aan4834.

16. Galley JD, Nelson MC, Yu Z, et al. Exposure to a social stressor disrupts the community structure of the colonic mucosa-associated microbiota. *BMC Microbiology.* 2014;14(1):189. https://doi.org/10.1186/1471-2180-14-189.

17. Added Sugar Repository. Hypoglycemia Support Foundation. Accessed February 15, 2023. https://hypoglycemia.org/added-sugar-repository/.

18. Kose J, Cheung A, Fezeu LK, et al. A comparison of sugar intake between individuals with high and low trait anxiety: Results from the NutriNet-Santé study. *Nutrients.* 2021;13(5):1526. https://doi.org/10.3390/nu13051526.

19. Di Rienzi SC, Britton RA. Adaptation of the gut microbiota to modern dietary sugars and sweeteners. *Advances in Nutrition.* 2019;11(3):616–29. https://doi.org/10.1093/advances/nmz118.

20. Daneman R, Prat A. The blood-brain barrier. *Cold Spring Harbor Perspectives in Biology.* 2015 Jan 5;7(1):a020412. https://doi.org/10.1101/cshperspect.a020412.

21. Chen Y, Xu J, Chen Y. Regulation of neurotransmitters by the gut microbiota and effects on cognition in neurological disorders. *Nutrients.* 2021;13(6):2099. https://doi.org/10.3390/nu13062099.

22. Terry N, Margolis KG. Serotonergic mechanisms regulating the GI tract: Experimental evidence and therapeutic relevance. *Gastrointestinal Pharmacology.* Published online. 2016:319–42. https://doi.org/10.1007/164_2016_103.

23. Kaur H, Bose C, Mande SS. Tryptophan metabolism by gut microbiome and gut-brain-axis: An *in silico* analysis. *Frontiers in Neuroscience.* 2019;13:1365. https://doi.org/10.3389/fnins.2019.01365.

24. Moncrieff J, Cooper RE, Stockmann T, et al. The serotonin theory of depression: A systematic umbrella review of the evidence. *Molecular Psychiatry.* 2022. https://doi.org/10.1038/s41380-022-01661-0.

25. Duranti S, Ruiz L, Lugli GA, et al. *Bifidobacterium adolescentis* as a key member of the human gut microbiota in the production of GABA. *Scientific Reports.* 2020;10(1). https://doi.org/10.1038/s41598-020-70986-z.

26. Simpson CA, Diaz-Arteche C, Eliby D, Schwartz OS, Simmons JG, Cowan CSM. The gut microbiota in anxiety and depression—a systematic review. *Clinical Psychology Review.* 2021;83:101943. https://doi.org/10.1016/j.cpr.2020.101943.

27. Clapp M, Aurora N, Herrera L, Bhatia M, Wilen E, Wakefield S. Gut microbiota's effect on mental health: The gut-brain axis. *Clinics and Practice.* 2017 Sep 15;7(4):987. https://doi.org/10.4081/cp.2017.987.

28. Silva YP, Bernardi A, Frozza RL. The role of short-chain fatty acids from gut microbiota in gut-brain communication. *Frontiers in Endocrinology.* 2020;11. https://doi.org/10.3389/fendo.2020.00025; Müller B, Rasmusson AJ, Just D, et al. Fecal short-chain fatty acid ratios as related to gastrointestinal and depressive symptoms in young adults. *Psychosomatic Medicine.* 2021 Sep 1;83(7):693–99. https://doi.org/10.1097/PSY.0000000000000965.

29. Yang B, Wei J, Ju P, Chen J. Effects of regulating intestinal microbiota on anxiety symptoms: A systematic review. *General Psychiatry.* 2019;32(2):e100056. https://doi.org/10.1136/gpsych-2019-100056.

Chapter 3: Immune to Anxiety

1. Wigren M, Nilsson J, Kaplan MJ. Pathogenic immunity in systemic lupus erythematosus and atherosclerosis: Common mechanisms and possible targets for intervention. *Journal of Internal Medicine.* 2015;278(5):494–506. https://doi.org/10.1111/joim.12357.

2. Guo M, Wang H, Xu S, et al. Alteration in gut microbiota is associated with dysregulation of cytokines and glucocorticoid therapy in systemic lupus erythematosus. *Gut Microbes.* 2020;11(6):1758–73. https://doi.org /10.1080/19490976.2020.1768644.

3. Ilchmann-Diounou H, Menard S. Psychological stress, intestinal barrier dysfunctions, and autoimmune disorders: An overview. *Frontiers in Immunology.* 2020 Aug 25;11:1823. https://doi.org/10.3389/fimmu.2020.01823.

4. Seiler A, Fagundes CP, Christian LM. The impact of everyday stressors on the immune system and health. In Choukèr A, ed. *Stress Challenges and Immunity in Space: From Mechanisms to Monitoring and Preventive Strategies.* Cham: Springer International Publishing; 2020:71–92. https://doi.org/10.1007 /978-3-030-16996-1_6.

5. Warrington R, Watson W, Kim HL, Antonetti FR. An introduction to immunology and immunopathology. *Allergy, Asthma, and Clinical Immunology.* 2011;7 Suppl 1(Suppl 1):S1. https://doi.org/10.1186/1710-1492-7-S1-S1.

6. Zhang JM, An J. Cytokines, inflammation, and pain. *International Anesthesiology Clinics.* 2007;45(2):27–37. https://doi.org/10.1097/aia.0b013e318 034194e.

7. Abel AM, Yang C, Thakar MS, Malarkannan S. Natural killer cells: Development, maturation, and clinical utilization. *Frontiers in Immunology.* 2018;9. https://doi.org/10.3389/fimmu.2018.01869.

8. Fowlkes A, Gaglani M, Groover K, et al. Effectiveness of COVID-19 vaccines in preventing SARS-CoV-2 infection among frontline workers before and during B.1.617.2 (Delta) variant predominance — eight U.S. locations, December 2020–August 2021. *Morbidity and Mortality Weekly Report.* 2021;70(34):1167–69. https://doi.org/10.15585/mmwr.mm7034e4.

9. Milani C, Duranti S, Bottacini F, et al. The first microbial colonizers of the human gut: Composition, activities, and health implications of the infant gut microbiota. *Microbiology and Molecular Biology Reviews.* 2017;81(4). https://doi.org/10.1128/mmbr.00036-17.

10. Reyman M, van Houten MA, van Baarle D, et al. Impact of delivery mode–associated gut microbiota dynamics on health in the first year of life. *Nature Communications.* 2019;10(1). https://doi.org/10.1038/s41467-019-13014-7.

11. van den Elsen LWJ, Garssen J, Burcelin R, Verhasselt V. Shaping the gut microbiota by breastfeeding: The gateway to allergy prevention? *Frontiers in Pediatrics*. 2019 Feb 27;7:47. https://doi.org/10.3389/fped.2019.00047.

12. Zhang H, Zhang Z, Liao Y, Zhang W, Tang D. The complex link and disease between the gut microbiome and the immune system in infants. *Frontiers in Cellular and Infection Microbiology*. 2022;12:924119. https://doi.org/10.3389/fcimb.2022.924119.

13. Borbet TC, Pawline MB, Zhang X, et al. Influence of the early-life gut microbiota on the immune responses to an inhaled allergen. *Mucosal Immunology*. 2022;15:1000–1011. https://doi.org/10.1038/s41385-022-00544-5.

14. de Goffau MC, Fuentes S, van den Bogert B, et al. Aberrant gut microbiota composition at the onset of type 1 diabetes in young children. *Diabetologia*. 2014;57(8):1569–77. https://doi.org/10.1007/s00125-014-3274-0.

15. Mahana D, Trent CM, Kurtz ZD, et al. Antibiotic perturbation of the murine gut microbiome enhances the adiposity, insulin resistance, and liver disease associated with high-fat diet. *Genome Medicine*. 2016;8(1):48. https://doi.org/10.1186/s13073-016-0297-9.

16. Carpay NC, Kamphorst K, de Meij TGJ, Daams JG, Vlieger AM, van Elburg RM. Microbial effects of prebiotics, probiotics and synbiotics after Caesarean section or exposure to antibiotics in the first week of life: A systematic review. *PLOS One*. 2022;17(11):e0277405. https://doi.org/10.1371/journal.pone.0277405.

17. Wiertsema SP, van Bergenhenegouwen J, Garssen J, Knippels LMJ. The interplay between the gut microbiome and the immune system in the context of infectious diseases throughout life and the role of nutrition in optimizing treatment strategies. *Nutrients*. 2021;13(3):886. https://doi.org/10.3390/nu13030886.

18. Okumura R, Takeda K. Roles of intestinal epithelial cells in the maintenance of gut homeostasis. *Experimental and Molecular Medicine*. 2017;49(5):e338. https://doi.org/10.1038/emm.2017.20.

19. Turner JR. Intestinal mucosal barrier function in health and disease. *Nature Reviews. Immunology*. 2009;9(11):799–809. https://doi.org/10.1038/nri2653.

20. Zheng D, Liwinski T, Elinav E. Interaction between microbiota and immunity in health and disease. *Cell Research*. 2020;30(6):492–506. https://doi.org/10.1038/s41422-020-0332-7.

21. Desai MS, Seekatz AM, Koropatkin NM, et al. A dietary fiber–deprived gut microbiota degrades the colonic mucus barrier and enhances pathogen susceptibility. *Cell*. 2016 Nov 17;167(5):1339–53.e21. https://doi.org/10.1016/j.cell.2016.10.043.

22. Bischoff SC, Barbara G, Buurman W, et al. Intestinal permeability—a new target for disease prevention and therapy. *BMC Gastroenterology.* 2014;14(1). https://doi.org/10.1186/s12876-014-0189-7.

23. Wang YH, Li JQ, Shi JF, et al. Depression and anxiety in relation to cancer incidence and mortality: A systematic review and meta-analysis of cohort studies. *Molecular Psychiatry.* 2020;25(7):1487–99. https://doi.org/10.1038/s41380-019-0595-x.

24. Alghamdi BS, Alatawi Y, Alshehri FS, Tayeb HO, Tarazi FI. Relationship between public mental health and immune status during the COVID-19 pandemic: Cross-sectional data from Saudi Arabia. *Risk Management and Healthcare Policy.* 2021 Apr 9;14:1439–47. https://doi.org/10.2147/RMHP.S302144.

25. Glaser R, Kiecolt-Glaser JK. Stress-induced immune dysfunction: Implications for health. *Nature Reviews. Immunology.* 2005;5(3):243–51. https://doi.org/10.1038/nri1571.

26. Dhabhar FS. The short-term stress response—mother nature's mechanism for enhancing protection and performance under conditions of threat, challenge, and opportunity. *Frontiers in Neuroendocrinology.* 2018;49:175–92. https://doi.org/10.1016/j.yfrne.2018.03.004.

27. Dhabhar FS. Enhancing versus suppressive effects of stress on immune function: Implications for immunoprotection and immunopathology. *Neuroimmunomodulation.* 2009;16(5):300–317. https://doi.org/10.1159/000216188.

28. Glaser R, Kiecolt-Glaser JK. Stress-induced immune dysfunction: Implications for health. *Nature Reviews. Immunology.* 2005;5(3):243–51. https://doi.org/10.1038/nri1571.

29. Segerstrom SC, Miller GE. Psychological stress and the human immune system: A meta-analytic study of 30 years of inquiry. *Psychological Bulletin.* 2004 Jul;130(4):601–30. https://doi.org/10.1037/0033-2909.130.4.601.

30. Bae YS, Shin EC, Bae YS, Van Eden W. Editorial: Stress and immunity. *Frontiers in Immunology.* 2019 Feb 14;10:245. https://doi.org/10.3389/fimmu.2019.00245.

31. Hou R, Garner M, Holmes C, et al. Peripheral inflammatory cytokines and immune balance in generalised anxiety disorder: Case-controlled study. *Brain, Behavior, and Immunity.* 2017;62:212–18. https://doi.org/10.1016/j.bbi.2017.01.021.

32. Wingo AP, Gibson G. Blood gene expression profiles suggest altered immune function associated with symptoms of generalized anxiety disorder. *Brain, Behavior, and Immunity.* 2015;43:184–91. https://doi.org/10.1016/j.bbi.2014.09.016.

33. Vieira MM, Ferreira TB, Pacheco PA, et al. Enhanced Th17 phenotype in individuals with generalized anxiety disorder. *Journal of Neuroimmunology.* 2010;229(1–2):212–18. https://doi.org/10.1016/j.jneuroim.2010.07.018.

34. Jeppesen R, Benros ME. Autoimmune diseases and psychotic disorders. *Frontiers in Psychiatry.* 2019;10. https://doi.org/10.3389/fpsyt.2019.00131.

35. Song H, Fang F, Tomasson G, et al. Association of stress-related disorders with subsequent autoimmune disease. JAMA. 2018;319(23):2388–2400. https://doi.org/10.1001/jama.2018.7028.

Chapter 4: Inflammation on the Brain

1. Manjunatha N, Ram D. Panic disorder in general medical practice—a narrative review. *Journal of Family Medicine and Primary Care.* 2022 Mar;11(3):861–69. https://doi.org/10.4103/jfmpc.jfmpc_888_21.

2. Kiecolt-Glaser JK. Stress, food, and inflammation: Psychoneuroimmunology and nutrition at the cutting edge. *Psychosomatic Medicine.* 2010 May;72(4):365–69. Epub April 21, 2010. https://doi.org/10.1097/PSY.0b013e3181dbf489.

3. Noncommunicable Diseases. World Health Organization. Accessed February 15, 2023. https://www.who.int/health-topics/noncommunicable-diseases#tab=tab_1.

4. Pahwa R, Goyal A, Jialal I. Chronic Inflammation. StatPearls. 2022:Jan–. Updated June 19, 2022. https://www.ncbi.nlm.nih.gov/books/NBK493173/.

5. Furman D, Campisi J, Verdin E, et al. Chronic inflammation in the etiology of disease across the life span. *Nature Medicine.* 2019;25(12):1822–32. https://doi.org/10.1038/s41591-019-0675-0.

6. Tanaka T, Narazaki M, Kishimoto T. IL-6 in inflammation, immunity, and disease. *Cold Spring Harbor Perspectives in Biology.* 2014 Sep 4;6(10):a016295. https://doi.org/10.1101/cshperspect.a016295. PMID: 25190079; PMCID: PMC4176007.

7. Chen L, Deng H, Cui H, et al. Inflammatory responses and inflammation-associated diseases in organs. *Oncotarget.* 2017 Dec 14;9(6):7204–18. https://doi.org/10.18632/oncotarget.23208. PMID: 29467962; PMCID: PMC5805548.

8. Renna ME, O'Toole MS, Spaeth PE, Lekander M, Mennin DS. The association between anxiety, traumatic stress, and obsessive-compulsive disorders and chronic inflammation: A systematic review and meta-analysis. *Depression and Anxiety.* 2018;35(11):1081–94. https://doi.org/10.1002/da.22790.

9. Costello H, Gould RL, Abrol E, Howard R. Systematic review and meta-analysis of the association between peripheral inflammatory cytokines and generalised anxiety disorder. *BMJ Open.* 2019;9(7):e027925. https://doi.org/10.1136/bmjopen-2018-027925.

10. Kennedy E, Niedzwiedz CL. The association of anxiety and stress-related disorders with C-reactive protein (CRP) within UK Biobank. *Brain, Behavior, and Immunity Health.* 2021;19:100410. https://doi.org/10.1016/j.bbih.2021 .100410.

11. Ye Z, Kappelmann N, Moser S, et al. Role of inflammation in depression and anxiety: Tests for disorder specificity, linearity and potential causality of association in the UK Biobank. *eClinicalMedicine.* 2021;38:100992. https://doi.org/10.1016/j.eclinm.2021.100992.

12. Osimo EF, Pillinger T, Rodriguez IM, Khandaker GM, Pariante CM, Howes OD. Inflammatory markers in depression: A meta-analysis of mean differences and variability in 5,166 patients and 5,083 controls. *Brain, Behavior, and Immunity.* 2020;87:901–9. https://doi.org/10.1016/j.bbi.2020.02.010.

13. Mesquita AR, Correia-Neves M, Roque S, et al. IL-10 modulates depressive-like behavior. *Journal of Psychiatric Research.* 2008;43(2):89–97. https://doi.org /10.1016/j.jpsychires.2008.02.004.

14. Dantzer R, O'Connor J, Freund G, et al. From inflammation to sickness and depression: When the immune system subjugates the brain. *Nature Reviews. Neuroscience.* 2008;9:46–56. https://doi.org/10.1038/nrn2297.

15. Liu YZ, Wang YX, Jiang CL. Inflammation: The common pathway of stress-related diseases. *Frontiers in Human Neuroscience.* 2017 Jun 20;11:316. https://doi.org/10.3389/fnhum.2017.00316.

16. Rohleder N. Stimulation of systemic low-grade inflammation by psychosocial stress. *Psychosomatic Medicine.* 2014;76(3):181–89. https://doi.org/10.1097 /PSY.0000000000000049.

17. Kiecolt-Glaser JK, McGuire L, Robles TF, Glaser R. Emotions, morbidity, and mortality: New perspectives from psychoneuroimmunology. *Annual Review of Psychology.* 2002;53:83–107. https://doi.org/10.1146/annurev.psych .53.100901.135217.

18. Glaser R, Robles TF, Sheridan J, Malarkey WB, Kiecolt-Glaser JK. Mild depressive symptoms are associated with amplified and prolonged inflammatory responses after influenza virus vaccination in older adults. *Archives of General Psychiatry.* 2003;60(10):1009–14. https://doi.org/10.1001/archpsyc .60.10.1009.

19. Felger JC. Imaging the role of inflammation in mood and anxiety-related disorders. *Current Neuropharmacology.* 2018;16(5):533–58. https://doi.org/1 0.2174/1570159X15666171123201142.

20. Michopoulos V, Powers A, Gillespie CF, Ressler KJ, Jovanovic T. Inflammation in fear- and anxiety-based disorders: PTSD, GAD, and beyond. *Neuropsychopharmacology.* 2017;42(1):254–70. https://doi.org/10.1038/npp.2016.146.

21. Hou R, Ye G, Liu Y, et al. Effects of SSRIs on peripheral inflammatory cytokines in patients with generalized anxiety disorder. *Brain, Behavior, and Immunity.* 2019;81:105–10. https://doi.org/10.1016/j.bbi.2019.06.001.

22. Hu K, Sjölander A, Lu D, et al. Aspirin and other non-steroidal anti-inflammatory drugs and depression, anxiety, and stress-related disorders following a cancer diagnosis: A nationwide register-based cohort study. *BMC Medicine.* 2020;18(1):238. https://doi.org/10.1186/s12916-020-01709-4.

23. DiSabato DJ, Quan N, Godbout JP. Neuroinflammation: The devil is in the details. *Journal of Neurochemistry.* 2016 Oct;139 Suppl 2(Suppl 2):136–53. https://doi.org/10.1111/jnc.13607.

24. Calcia MA, Bonsall DR, Bloomfield PS, Selvaraj S, Barichello T, Howes OD. Stress and neuroinflammation: A systematic review of the effects of stress on microglia and the implications for mental illness. *Psychopharmacology.* 2016;233(9):1637–50. https://doi.org/10.1007/s00213-016-4218-9.

25. León-Rodríguez A, Fernández-Arjona M del M, Grondona JM, Pedraza C, López-Ávalos MD. Anxiety-like behavior and microglial activation in the amygdala after acute neuroinflammation induced by microbial neuraminidase. *Scientific Reports.* 2022;12(1). https://doi.org/10.1038/s41598-022-15617-5.

26. Wang H, He Y, Sun Z, et al. Microglia in depression: An overview of microglia in the pathogenesis and treatment of depression. *Journal of Neuroinflammation.* 2022;19(1). https://doi.org/10.1186/s12974-022-02492-0.

27. Bachiller S, Jiménez-Ferrer I, Paulus A, et al. Microglia in neurological diseases: A road map to brain-disease dependent-inflammatory response. *Frontiers in Cellular Neuroscience.* 2018;12.

28. Fontana L, Ghezzi L, Cross AH, Piccio L. Effects of dietary restriction on neuroinflammation in neurodegenerative diseases. *Journal of Experimental Medicine.* 2021;218(2):e20190086. https://doi.org/10.1084/jem.20190086.

29. Zhou L, Chen L, Li X, Li T, Dong Z, Wang YT. Food allergy induces alteration in brain inflammatory status and cognitive impairments. *Behavioural Brain Research.* 2019;364:374–82. https://doi.org/10.1016/j.bbr.2018.01.011.

30. Gupta RS, Warren CM, Smith BM, et al. Prevalence and severity of food allergies among US adults. *JAMA Network Open.* 2019;2(1):e185630. https://doi.org/10.1001/jamanetworkopen.2018.5630.

31. Bunyavanich S, Berin MC. Food allergy and the microbiome: Current understandings and future directions. *Journal of Allergy and Clinical Immunology.* 2019 Dec;144(6):1468–77. https://doi.org/10.1016/j.jaci.2019.10.019. PMID: 31812181; PMCID: PMC6905201.

32. Bolte LA, Vich Vila A, Imhann F, et al. Long-term dietary patterns are associated with pro-inflammatory and anti-inflammatory features of the gut

microbiome. *Gut.* 2021;70(7):1287–98. https://doi.org/10.1136/gutjnl-2020 -322670.

Chapter 5: Anxiety and Leptin, the Appetite Hormone

1. van Strien T, Gibson EL, Baños R, Cebolla A, Winkens LHH. Is comfort food actually comforting for emotional eaters? A (moderated) mediation analysis. *Physiology and Behavior.* 2019;211:112671. https://doi.org/10.1016/j .physbeh.2019.112671.

2. Cinti F, Cinti S. The endocrine adipose organ: A system playing a central role in COVID-19. *Cells.* 2022;11(13):2109. https://doi.org/10.3390/cells11132109.

3. Bouillon-Minois JB, Trousselard M, Thivel D, et al. Leptin as a biomarker of stress: A systematic review and meta-analysis. *Nutrients.* 2021;13(10):3350. https://doi.org/10.3390/nu13103350.

4. Tomiyama AJ, Schamarek I, Lustig RH, et al. Leptin concentrations in response to acute stress predict subsequent intake of comfort foods. *Physiology and Behavior.* 2012;107(1):34–39. https://doi.org/10.1016/j.physbeh.2012 .04.021.

5. Gruzdeva O, Borodkina D, Uchasova E, Dyleva Y, Barbarash O. Leptin resistance: Underlying mechanisms and diagnosis. *Diabetes, Metabolic Syndrome and Obesity: Targets and Therapy.* 2019 Jan 25;12:191–98. https://doi .org/10.2147/DMSO.S182406.

6. Misch M, Puthanveetil P. The head-to-toe hormone: Leptin as an extensive modulator of physiologic systems. *International Journal of Molecular Sciences.* 2022;23(10):5439. https://doi.org/10.3390/ijms23105439.

7. Côté I, Green SM, Toklu HZ, et al. Differential physiological responses to central leptin overexpression in male and female rats. *Journal of Neuroendocrinology.* 2017 Dec;29(12):10.1111/jne.12552. https://doi.org/10.1111/jne .12552.

8. Behre HM, Simoni M, Nieschlag E. Strong association between serum levels of leptin and testosterone in men. *Clinical Endocrinology.* 1997;47(2): 237–40. https://doi.org/10.1046/j.1365-2265.1997.2681067.x.

9. Van Harmelen V, Reynisdottir S, Eriksson P, et al. Leptin secretion from subcutaneous and visceral adipose tissue in women. *Diabetes.* 1998;47(6): 913–17. https://doi.org/10.2337/diabetes.47.6.913.

10. Dornbush S, Aeddula NR. Physiology, Leptin. StatPearls. 2022. Accessed October 14, 2022. http://www.ncbi.nlm.nih.gov/books/NBK537038/.

11. Wang W, Liu S, Li K, et al. Leptin: A potential anxiolytic by facilitation of fear extinction. *CNS Neuroscience and Therapeutics.* 2015;21(5):425–34. https://doi.org/10.1111/cns.12375; Liu J, Garza JC, Bronner J, Kim CS, Zhang

W, Lu XY. Acute administration of leptin produces anxiolytic-like effects: A comparison with fluoxetine. *Psychopharmacology.* 2010;207(4):535–45. https://doi.org/10.1007/s00213-009-1684-3.

12. Gold PW. Endocrine factors in key structural and intracellular changes in depression. *Trends in Endocrinology and Metabolism.* 2021;32(4):212–23. https://doi.org/10.1016/j.tem.2021.01.003; Lawson EA, Miller KK, Blum JI, et al. Leptin levels are associated with decreased depressive symptoms in women across the weight spectrum, independent of body fat. *Clinical Endocrinology.* 2012;76(4):520–25. https://doi.org/10.1111/j.1365-2265.2011.04182.x.

13. https://www.accessdata.fda.gov/drugsatfda_docs/label/2017/209637lbl.pdf.

14. https://pubmed.ncbi.nlm.nih.gov/19853906/.

15. Masdrakis VG, Papageorgiou C, Markianos M. Associations of plasma leptin to clinical manifestations in reproductive aged female patients with panic disorder. *Psychiatry Research.* 2017;255:161–66. https://doi.org/10.1016/j.psychres.2017.05.025.

16. Salerno PSV, Bastos CR, Peres A, et al. Leptin polymorphism rs3828942: Risk for anxiety disorders? *European Archives of Psychiatry and Clinical Neuroscience.* Published online August 16, 2019. https://doi.org/10.1007/s00406-019-01051-8.

17. Atmaca M, Tezcan E, Kuloglu M, Ustundag B. Serum leptin levels in obsessive-compulsive disorder. *Psychiatry and Clinical Neurosciences.* 2005;59(2):189–93. https://doi.org/10.1111/j.1440-1819.2005.01356.x.

18. Lei Y, Wang D, Bai Y, et al. Leptin enhances social motivation and reverses chronic unpredictable stress-induced social anhedonia during adolescence. *Molecular Psychiatry.* Published online September 22, 2022. https://doi.org/10.1038/s41380-022-01778-2.

19. Renna ME, Shrout MR, Madison AA, et al. Fluctuations in depression and anxiety predict dysregulated leptin among obese breast cancer survivors. *Journal of Cancer Survivorship.* 2021;15(6):847–54. https://doi.org/10.1007/s11764-020-00977-6.

20. Byrne ME, Tanofsky-Kraff M, Jaramillo M, et al. Relationships of trait anxiety and loss of control eating with serum leptin concentrations among youth. *Nutrients.* 2019;11(9):2198. https://doi.org/10.3390/nu11092198.

21. Farr OM, Ko BJ, Joung KE, et al. Posttraumatic stress disorder, alone or additively with early life adversity, is associated with obesity and cardiometabolic risk. *Nutrition, Metabolism, and Cardiovascular Diseases.* 2015;25(5):479–88. https://doi.org/10.1016/j.numecd.2015.01.007.

22. Changchien TC, Tai CM, Huang CK, Chien CC, Yen YC. Psychiatric symptoms and leptin in obese patients who were bariatric surgery candi-

dates. *Neuropsychiatric Disease and Treatment.* 2015;11:2153–58. https://doi .org/10.2147/NDT.S88075.

23. Wang J, Obici S, Morgan K, Barzilai N, Feng Z, Rossetti L. Overfeeding rapidly induces leptin and insulin resistance. *Diabetes.* 2001;50(12):2786–91. https://doi.org/10.2337/diabetes.50.12.2786.

24. Enriori PJ, Evans AE, Sinnayah P, et al. Diet-induced obesity causes severe but reversible leptin resistance in arcuate melanocortin neurons. *Cell Metabolism.* 2007;5(3):181–94. https://doi.org/10.1016/j.cmet.2007.02.004.

25. Mendoza-Herrera K, Florio AA, Moore M, et al. The leptin system and diet: A mini review of the current evidence. *Frontiers in Endocrinology.* 2021;12:749050. https://doi.org/10.3389/fendo.2021.749050.

26. Shapiro A, Tümer N, Gao Y, Cheng KY, Scarpace PJ. Prevention and reversal of diet-induced leptin resistance with a sugar-free diet despite high fat content. *British Journal of Nutrition.* 2011;106(3):390–97. https://doi .org/10.1017/S000711451100033X.

27. Spruijt-Metz D, Belcher B, Anderson D, et al. A high-sugar/low-fiber meal compared with a low-sugar/high-fiber meal leads to higher leptin and physical activity levels in overweight Latina females. *Journal of the American Dietetic Association.* 2009 Jun;109(6):1058–63. https://doi.org/10.1016/j.jada.2009.03.013.

Chapter 6: The Dangers of Metabolic Disruption

1. Grigsby AB, Anderson RJ, Freedland KE, Clouse RE, Lustman PJ. Prevalence of anxiety in adults with diabetes: A systematic review. *Journal of Psychosomatic Research.* 2002;53(6):1053–60. https://doi.org/10.1016/s0022 -3999(02)00417-8.

2. Li C, Barker L, Ford ES, Zhang X, Strine TW, Mokdad AH. Diabetes and anxiety in US adults: Findings from the 2006 Behavioral Risk Factor Surveillance System. *Diabetic Medicine.* 2008;25(7):878–81. https://doi.org/10 .1111/j.1464-5491.2008.02477.x.

3. Khuwaja AK, Lalani S, Dhanani R, Azam IS, Rafique G, White F. Anxiety and depression among outpatients with type 2 diabetes: A multi-centre study of prevalence and associated factors. *Diabetology and Metabolic Syndrome.* 2010;2(1):72. https://doi.org/10.1186/1758-5996-2-72.

4. Grigsby AB, Anderson RJ, Freedland KE, Clouse RE, Lustman PJ. Prevalence of anxiety in adults with diabetes: A systematic review. *Journal of Psychosomatic Research.* 2002;53(6):1053–60. https://doi.org/10.1016/s0022-3999(02)00417-8.

5. Esposito K, Giugliano D. The metabolic syndrome and inflammation: Association or causation? *Nutrition, Metabolism and Cardiovascular Diseases.* 2004;14(5):228–32. https://doi.org/10.1016/s0939-4753(04)80048-6.

6. Araújo J, Cai J, Stevens J. Prevalence of optimal metabolic health in American adults: National Health and Nutrition Examination Survey 2009–2016. *Metabolic Syndrome and Related Disorders*. 2019;17(1):46–52. https://doi .org/10.1089/met.2018.0105.

7. Hirode G, Wong RJ. Trends in the prevalence of metabolic syndrome in the United States, 2011–2016. *JAMA*. 2020;323(24):2526–28. https://doi .org/10.1001/jama.2020.4501.

8. National Diabetes Statistics Report. Centers for Disease Control and Prevention. https://www.cdc.gov/diabetes/data/statistics-report/index.html. Accessed January 10, 2023.

9. Humer E, Pieh C, Probst T. Metabolomic biomarkers in anxiety disorders. *International Journal of Molecular Sciences*. 2020;21(13):4784. https://doi .org/10.3390/ijms21134784.

10. Peter H, Goebel P, Müller S, Hand I. Clinically relevant cholesterol elevation in anxiety disorders: A comparison with normal controls. *International Journal of Behavioral Medicine*. 1999;6(1):30–39. https://doi.org/10.1207 /s15327558ijbm0601_3.

11. Han A. Association between lipid ratio and depression: A cross-sectional study. *Scientific Reports*. 2022;12:6190. https://doi.org/10.1038/s41598-022-10350-5.

12. Cruz JN da, Magro DDD, Lima DD de, Cruz JGP da. Simvastatin treatment reduces the cholesterol content of membrane/lipid rafts, implicating the N-methyl-D-aspartate receptor in anxiety: A literature review. *Brazilian Journal of Pharmaceutical Sciences*. 2017;53(1). https://doi.org/10.1590/s2175 -97902017000116102.

13. Koorneef LL, Bogaards M, Reinders MJT, Meijer OC, Mahfouz A. How metabolic state may regulate fear: Presence of metabolic receptors in the fear circuitry. *Frontiers in Neuroscience*. 2018;12:594. https://doi.org/10.3389 /fnins.2018.00594.

14. Kahl KG, Schweiger U, Correll C, et al. Depression, anxiety disorders, and metabolic syndrome in a population at risk for type 2 diabetes mellitus. *Brain and Behavior*. 2015;5(3):e00306. https://doi.org/10.1002/brb3.306.

15. Gariepy G, Nitka D, Schmitz N. The association between obesity and anxiety disorders in the population: A systematic review and meta-analysis. *International Journal of Obesity*. 2010;34(3):407–19. https://doi.org/10.1038 /ijo.2009.252.

16. Labenz C, Huber Y, Michel M, et al. Nonalcoholic fatty liver disease increases the risk of anxiety and depression. *Hepatology Communications*. 2020;4(9):1293–1301. https://doi.org/10.1002/hep4.1541.

17. Bouayed J, Rammal H, Soulimani R. Oxidative stress and anxiety: Relationship and cellular pathways. *Oxidative Medicine and Cellular Longevity.* 2009 Apr–Jun;2(2):63–67. https://doi.org/10.4161/oxim.2.2.7944. PMID: 20357926; PMCID: PMC2763246.

18. Ryan KK. *Stress and Metabolic Disease.* Washington, DC: National Academies Press; 2014. Accessed October 31, 2022. https://www.ncbi.nlm.nih.gov /books/NBK242443/.

19. de Kluiver H, Jansen R, Milaneschi Y, et al. Metabolomic profiles discriminating anxiety from depression. *Acta Psychiatrica Scandinavica.* 2021;144(2):178–93. https://doi.org/10.1111/acps.13310.

20. Needham BD, Funabashi M, Adame MD, et al. A gut-derived metabolite alters brain activity and anxiety behaviour in mice. *Nature.* 2022;602(7898): 647–53. https://doi.org/10.1038/s41586-022-04396-8.

21. Martin AM, Sun EW, Rogers GB, Keating DJ. The influence of the gut microbiome on host metabolism through the regulation of gut hormone release. *Frontiers in Physiology.* 2019;10:428. https://doi.org/10.3389/fphys.2019.00428.

22. Vernocchi P, Del Chierico F, Putignani L. Gut microbiota metabolism and interaction with food components. *International Journal of Molecular Sciences.* 2020 May 23;21(10):3688. https://doi.org/10.3390/ijms21103688; Fan Y, Pedersen O. Gut microbiota in human metabolic health and disease. *Nature Reviews. Microbiology.* 2021;19(1):55–71. https://doi.org/10.1038/s41579 -020-0433-9.

23. Fukao A, Takamatsu J, Arishima T, et al. Graves' disease and mental disorders. *Journal of Clinical and Translational Endocrinology.* 2020;19. https:// doi.org/10.1016/j.jcte.2019.100207.

24. Vásquez-Alvarez S, Bustamante-Villagomez SK, Vazquez-Marroquin G, et al. Metabolic age, an index based on basal metabolic rate, can predict individuals that are high risk of developing metabolic syndrome. *High Blood Pressure and Cardiovascular Prevention.* 2021;28(3):263–70. https://doi.org /10.1007/s40292-021-00441-1.

25. Troisi A, Moles A, Panepuccia L, Lo Russo D, Palla G, Scucchi S. Serum cholesterol levels and mood symptoms in the postpartum period. *Psychiatry Research.* 2002;109(3):213–19. https://doi.org/10.1016/s0165-1781(02)00020-3.

Chapter 7: Macronutrients

1. La Berge AF. How the ideology of low fat conquered America. *Journal of the History of Medicine and Allied Sciences.* 2008;63(2):139–77. https://doi .org/10.1093/jhmas/jrn001.

2. Oh R, Gilani B, Uppaluri KR. Low Carbohydrate Diet. StatPearls. July 11, 2022. https://www.ncbi.nlm.nih.gov/books/NBK537084/.

3. Wheatley SD, Deakin TA, Arjomandkhah NC, Hollinrake PB, Reeves TE. Low carbohydrate dietary approaches for people with type 2 diabetes—a narrative review. *Frontiers in Nutrition.* 2021;8:687658. https://doi.org/10.3389 /fnut.2021.687658.

4. Wright N, Wilson L, Smith M, Duncan B, McHugh P. The BROAD study: A randomised controlled trial using a whole food plant-based diet in the community for obesity, ischaemic heart disease or diabetes. *Nutrition and Diabetes.* 2017;7(3):e256. https://doi.org/10.1038/nutd.2017.3.

5. Chang CY, Ke DS, Chen JY. Essential fatty acids and human brain. *Acta Neurologica Taiwanica.* 2009;18(4):231–41.

6. Ventriglio A, Sancassiani F, Contu MP, et al. Mediterranean diet and its benefits on health and mental health: A literature review. *Clinical Practice and Epidemiology in Mental Health.* 2020 Jul 30;16(Suppl 1):156–64. https:// doi.org/10.2174/1745017902016010156.

7. Machate DJ, Figueiredo PS, Marcelino G, et al. Fatty acid diets: Regulation of gut microbiota composition and obesity and its related metabolic dysbiosis. *International Journal of Molecular Sciences.* 2020 Jun 8;21(11):4093. https://doi.org/10.3390/ijms21114093.

8. Rocha DM, Bressan J, Hermsdorff HH. The role of dietary fatty acid intake in inflammatory gene expression: A critical review. *Sao Paulo Medical Journal.* 2017;135(2):157–68. https://doi.org/10.1590/1516-3180.2016 .008607072016.

9. Sheashea M, Xiao J, Farag MA. MUFA in metabolic syndrome and associated risk factors: Is MUFA the opposite side of the PUFA coin? *Food and Function.* 2021;12(24):12221–34. https://doi.org/10.1039/d1fo00979f.

10. Fatemi F, Siassi F, Qorbani M, Sotoudeh G. Higher dietary fat quality is associated with lower anxiety score in women: A cross-sectional study. *Annals of General Psychiatry.* 2020 Feb 26;19:14. https://doi.org/10.1186/s12991 -020-00264-9. PMID: 32127909; PMCID: PMC7045483.

11. Wolfe AR, Ogbonna EM, Lim S, Li Y, Zhang J. Dietary linoleic and oleic fatty acids in relation to severe depressed mood: 10 years follow-up of a national cohort. *Progress in Neuro-Psychopharmacology and Biological Psychiatry.* 2009;33(6):972–77. https://doi.org/10.1016/j.pnpbp.2009.05.002.

12. Innes JK, Calder PC. Omega-6 fatty acids and inflammation. *Prostaglandins, Leukotrienes and Essential Fatty Acids.* 2018;132:41–48. https://doi.org/10.1016/j .plefa.2018.03.004.

13. DiNicolantonio JJ, O'Keefe JH. The importance of marine omega-3s for brain development and the prevention and treatment of behavior, mood, and other brain disorders. *Nutrients.* 2020 Aug 4;12(8):2333. https://doi.org /10.3390/nu12082333.

14. Su KP, Tseng PT, Lin PY, et al. Association of use of omega-3 polyunsaturated fatty acids with changes in severity of anxiety symptoms: A systematic review and meta-analysis. *JAMA Network Open.* 2018 Sep 7;1(5):e182327. https://doi.org/10.1001/jamanetworkopen.2018.2327; Yang R, Wang L, Jin K, et al. Omega-3 polyunsaturated fatty acids supplementation alleviate anxiety rather than depressive symptoms among first-diagnosed, drug-naïve major depressive disorder patients: A randomized clinical trial. *Frontiers in Nutrition.* 2022 Jul 12;9:876152; Su KP, Tseng PT, Lin PY, et al. Association of use of omega-3 polyunsaturated fatty acids with changes in severity of anxiety symptoms: A systematic review and meta-analysis. *JAMA Network Open.* 2018 Sep 7;1(5):e182327. https://doi.org/10.1001/jamanetworkopen .2018.2327; Polokowski AR, Shakil H, Carmichael CL, Reigada LC. Omega-3 fatty acids and anxiety: A systematic review of the possible mechanisms at play. *Nutritional Neuroscience.* 2018;23(7):494–504. https:// doi.org/10.1080/1028415x.2018.1525092.

15. 7 Things to Know about Omega-3 Fatty Acids. National Center for Complementary and Integrative Health. https://www.nccih.nih.gov/health/tips /things-to-know-about-omega-fatty-acids.

16. Simopoulos AP. The importance of the ratio of omega-6/omega-3 essential fatty acids. *Biomedicine and Pharmacotherapy.* 2002;56(8):365–79. https:// doi.org/10.1016/s0753-3322(02)00253-6.

17. Yehuda S, Rabinovitz S, Mostofsky DI. Mixture of essential fatty acids lowers test anxiety. *Nutritional Neuroscience.* 2005;8(4):265–67. https://doi .org/10.1080/10284150500445795.

18. Nakajima S, Fukasawa K, Gotoh M, Murakami-Murofushi K, Kunugi H. Saturated fatty acid is a principal cause of anxiety-like behavior in diet-induced obese rats in relation to serum lysophosphatidyl choline level. *International Journal of Obesity.* 2020;44(3):727–38. https://doi.org/10.1038 /s41366-019-0468-z.

19. Melo HM, Santos LE, Ferreira ST. Diet-derived fatty acids, brain inflammation, and mental health. *Frontiers in Neuroscience.* 2019 Mar 26;13:265. https://doi.org/10.3389/fnins.2019.00265.

20. Astrup A, Magkos F, Bier DM, et al. Saturated fats and health: A reassessment and proposal for food-based recommendations. *Journal of the American*

College of Cardiology. 2020;76(7):844–57. https://doi.org/10.1016/j.jacc.2020 .05.077.

21. Dhaka V, Gulia N, Ahlawat KS, Khatkar BS. Trans fats—sources, health risks and alternative approach—a review. *Journal of Food Science and Technology.* 2011 Oct;48(5):534–41. https://doi.org/10.1007/s13197-010-0225-8.

22. Mozaffarian D. Trans fatty acids—effects on systemic inflammation and endothelial function. *Atherosclerosis Supplements.* 2006;7(2):29–32. https://doi.org/10.1016/j.atherosclerosissup.2006.04.007.

23. Pase CS, Roversi K, Trevizol F, et al. Influence of perinatal trans fat on behavioral responses and brain oxidative status of adolescent rats acutely exposed to stress. *Neuroscience.* 2013;247:242–52. https://doi.org/10.1016/j.neuroscience.2013.05.053; Meichtry LB, Poetini MR, Dahleh MMM, et al. Addition of saturated and trans-fatty acids to the diet induces depressive and anxiety-like behaviors in drosophila melanogaster. *Neuroscience.* 2020;443:164–75.

24. Hashemi S, Amani R, Cheraghian B, Neamatpour S. Stress and anxiety levels are associated with erythrocyte fatty acids content in young women. *Iranian Journal of Psychiatry.* 2020 Jan;15(1):47–54. PMID: 32377214; PMCID: PMC7193237; Ford PA, Jaceldo-Siegl K, Lee JW, Tonstad S. Trans fatty acid intake is related to emotional affect in the Adventist Health Study-2. *Nutrition Research.* 2016 Jun;36(6):509–17. https://doi.org/10.1016/j.nutres.2016.01.005;2.

25. Aucoin M, LaChance L, Naidoo U, et al. Diet and anxiety: A scoping review. *Nutrients.* 2021 Dec 10;13(12):4418. https://doi.org/10.3390/nu13124418. PMID: 34959972; PMCID: PMC8706568.

26. Aucoin M, Bhardwaj S. Generalized anxiety disorder and hypoglycemia symptoms improved with diet modification. *Case Reports in Psychiatry.* 2016;2016:7165425. https://doi.org/10.1155/2016/7165425.

27. Gangwisch JE, Hale L, Garcia L, et al. High glycemic index diet as a risk factor for depression: Analyses from the Women's Health Initiative. *American Journal of Clinical Nutrition.* 2015 Aug;102(2):454–63. https://doi.org/10.3945/ajcn.114.103846.

28. Kim Y, Chen J, Wirth MD, Shivappa N, Hebert JR. Lower dietary inflammatory index scores are associated with lower glycemic index scores among college students. *Nutrients.* 2018 Feb 7;10(2):182. https://doi.org/10.3390/nu10020182.

29. Campbell GJ, Senior AM, Bell-Anderson KS. Metabolic effects of high glycaemic index diets: A systematic review and meta-analysis of feeding studies in mice and rats. *Nutrients.* 2017 Jun 22;9(7):646. https://doi.org/10.3390/nu9070646.

30. Saghafian F, Sharif N, Saneei P, et al. Consumption of dietary fiber in relation to psychological disorders in adults. *Frontiers in Psychiatry.* 2021 Jun 24;12:587468. https://doi.org/10.3389/fpsyt.2021.587468.

Notes

31. Swann OG, Kilpatrick M, Breslin M, Oddy WH. Dietary fiber and its associations with depression and inflammation. *Nutrition Reviews.* 2020;78(5):394–411. https://doi.org/10.1093/nutrit/nuz072.

32. Brown L, Rosner B, Willett WW, Sacks FM. Cholesterol-lowering effects of dietary fiber: A meta-analysis. *American Journal of Clinical Nutrition.* 1999;69(1):30–42. https://doi.org/10.1093/ajcn/69.1.30.

33. Carlson JL, Erickson JM, Lloyd BB, Slavin JL. Health effects and sources of prebiotic dietary fiber. *Current Developments in Nutrition.* 2018 Jan 29;2(3):nzy005. https://doi.org/10.1093/cdn/nzy005. PMID: 30019028; PMCID: PMC6041804.

34. Myhrstad MCW, Tunsjø H, Charnock C, Telle-Hansen VH. Dietary fiber, gut microbiota, and metabolic regulation—current status in human randomized trials. *Nutrients.* 2020 Mar 23;12(3):859. https://doi.org/10.3390/nu12030859.

35. Fiber. The Nutrition Source. Harvard T.H. Chan School of Public Health. Accessed February 16, 2023. https://www.hsph.harvard.edu/nutritionsource/carbohydrates/fiber/.

36. Kose J, Cheung A, Fezeu LK, et al. A comparison of sugar intake between individuals with high and low trait anxiety: Results from the NutriNet-Santé study. *Nutrients.* 2021 Apr 30;13(5):1526. https://doi.org/10.3390/nu13051526. PMID: 33946586; PMCID: PMC8147234.

37. Westover AN, Marangell LB. A cross-national relationship between sugar consumption and major depression? *Depression and Anxiety.* 2002;16(3):118–20. https://doi.org/10.1002/da.10054.

38. Alam YH, Kim R, Jang C. Metabolism and health impacts of dietary sugars. *Journal of Lipid and Atherosclerosis.* 2022;11(1):20–38. https://doi.org/10.12997/jla.2022.11.1.20.

39. Satokari R. High intake of sugar and the balance between pro- and anti-inflammatory gut bacteria. *Nutrients.* 2020 May 8;12(5):1348. https://doi.org/10.3390/nu12051348.

40. Jacques A, Chaaya N, Beecher K, Ali SA, Belmer A, Bartlett S. The impact of sugar consumption on stress driven, emotional and addictive behaviors. *Neuroscience and Biobehavioral Reviews.* 2019;103:178–99. https://doi.org/10.1016/j.neubiorev.2019.05.021.

41. https://www.who.int/news/item/14-07-2023-aspartame-hazard-and-risk-assessment-results-released.

42. Okasha EF. Effect of long term-administration of aspartame on the ultra-structure of sciatic nerve. *Journal of Microscopy and Ultrastructure.* 2016 Oct–Dec;4(4):175–83. https://doi.org/10.1016/j.jmau.2016.02.001.

43. Choudhary AK, Lee YY. Neurophysiological symptoms and aspartame: What is the connection? *Nutrition Neuroscience.* 2018;21(5):306–16. https:// doi.org/10.1080/1028415X.2017.1288340.

44. Norwitz NG, Naidoo U. Nutrition as metabolic treatment for anxiety. *Frontiers in Psychiatry.* 2021;12. https://doi.org/10.3389/fpsyt.2021.598119.

45. de Lorgeril M, Salen P. Gluten and wheat intolerance today: Are modern wheat strains involved? *International Journal of Food Sciences and Nutrition.* 2014;65(5):577–81. https://doi.org/10.3109/09637486.2014.886185.

46. Clappison E, Hadjivassiliou M, Zis P. Psychiatric manifestations of coeliac disease, a systematic review and meta-analysis. *Nutrients.* 2020;12(1):142. https://doi.org/10.3390/nu12010142.

47. Casella G, Pozzi R, Cigognetti M, et al. Mood disorders and non-celiac gluten sensitivity. *Minerva Gastroenterology.* 2017;63(1):32–37. https://doi .org/10.23736/S1121-421X.16.02325-4.

48. Khanna P, Aeri BT. Association of quantity and quality of protein intake with depression and anxiety symptoms among adolescent boys and girls (13–15 years) studying in public schools of Delhi. *Journal of Nutritional Science and Vitaminology.* 2020;66(Supp):S141–S148. https://doi.org/10.3177/jnsv.66.S141.

49. Leitzmann C. Vegetarian nutrition: Past, present, future. *American Journal of Clinical Nutrition.* 2014;100 Suppl 1:496S–502S. https://doi.org/10.3945 /ajcn.113.071365.

50. Forgrieve J. The Growing Acceptance of Veganism. *Forbes.* November 2, 2018. https://www.forbes.com/sites/janetforgrieve/2018/11/02/picturing-a -kindler-gentler-world-vegan-month/?sh=44639a4f2f2b.

51. Varian E. It's called "plant-based," look it up. *New York Times.* December 28, 2019. https://www.nytimes.com/2019/12/28/style/plant-based-diet.html.

52. Dobersek U, Teel K, Altmeyer S, Adkins J, Wy G, Peak J. Meat and mental health: A meta-analysis of meat consumption, depression, and anxiety. Published online ahead of print, October 6, 2021. *Critical Reviews in Food Science and Nutrition.* 2021;1–18. https://doi.org/10.1080/10408398.2021.1 974336.

53. Beezhold B, Radnitz C, Rinne A, DiMatteo J. Vegans report less stress and anxiety than omnivores. *Nutritional Neuroscience.* 2015;18(7):289–96. https://doi.org/10.1179/1476830514Y.0000000164.

54. Bègue L, Shankland R. Is vegetarianism related to anxiety and depression? A cross-sectional survey in a French sample. *Journal of Health, Population and Nutrition.* 2022;41(18). https://doi.org/10.1186/s41043-022-00300-2.

55. Lee MF, Eather R, Best T. Plant-based dietary quality and depressive symptoms in Australian vegans and vegetarians: A cross-sectional study. *BMJ*

Nutrition, Prevention and Health. 2021;e000332. https://doi.org/10.1136 /bmjnph-2021-000332.

56. Jenkins TA, Nguyen JC, Polglaze KE, Bertrand PP. Influence of tryptophan and serotonin on mood and cognition with a possible role of the gut-brain axis. *Nutrients.* 2016 Jan 20;8(1):56. https://doi.org/10.3390/nu8010056.

57. Lindseth G, Helland B, Caspers J. The effects of dietary tryptophan on affective disorders. *Archives of Psychiatric Nursing.* 2015 Apr;29(2):102–7. https://doi.org/10.1016/j.apnu.2014.11.008.

58. Wurtman RJ, Hefti F, Melamed E. Precursor control of neurotransmitter synthesis. *Pharmacological Reviews.* 1980;32(4):315–35.

59. Hudson C, Hudson S, MacKenzie J. Protein-source tryptophan as an efficacious treatment for social anxiety disorder: A pilot study. *Canadian Journal of Physiology and Pharmacology.* 2007;85(9):928–32. https://doi.org/10.1139 /Y07-082.

60. Schopman SME, Bosman RC, Muntingh ADT, et al. Effects of tryptophan depletion on anxiety, a systematic review. *Translational Psychiatry.* 2021;11(118). https://doi.org/10.1038/s41398-021-01219-8.

61. Zanfirescu A, Ungurianu A, Tsatsakis AM, et al. A review of the alleged health hazards of monosodium glutamate [published correction appears in *Comprehensive Reviews in Food Science and Food Safety.* 2020 Jul;19(4):2330]. *Comprehensive Reviews in Food Science and Food Safety.* 2019;18(4):1111–34. https://doi.org/10.1111/1541-4337.12448.

62. Nasir M, Trujillo D, Levine J, Dwyer JB, Rupp ZW, Bloch MH. Glutamate systems in DSM-5 anxiety disorders: Their role and a review of glutamate and GABA psychopharmacology. *Frontiers in Psychiatry.* 2020;11:548505.

63. Onaolapo OJ, Aremu OS, Onaolapo AY. Monosodium glutamate-associated alterations in open field, anxiety-related and conditioned place preference behaviours in mice. *Naunyn-Schmiedeberg's Archives of Pharmacology.* 2017;390(7):677–89. https://doi.org/10.1007/s00210-017-1371-6.

64. Banerjee A, Mukherjee S, Maji BK. Worldwide flavor enhancer monosodium glutamate combined with high lipid diet provokes metabolic alterations and systemic anomalies: An overview. *Toxicology Reports.* 2021;8:938–61. https://doi.org/10.1016/j.toxrep.2021.04.009.

Chapter 8: Micronutrients

1. Lopresti AL. The effects of psychological and environmental stress on micronutrient concentrations in the body: A review of the evidence. *Advances in Nutrition.* 2020;11(1):103–12. https://doi.org/10.1093/advances /nmz082.

2. Petroski W, Minich DM. Is there such a thing as "anti-nutrients"? A narrative review of perceived problematic plant compounds. *Nutrients.* 2020 Sep 24;12(10):2929. https://doi.org/10.3390/nu12102929.

3. Schlemmer U, Frølich W, Prieto RM, Grases F. Phytate in foods and significance for humans: Food sources, intake, processing, bioavailability, protective role and analysis. *Molecular Nutrition and Food Research.* 2009;53 Suppl 2:S330–S375. https://doi.org/10.1002/mnfr.200900099.

4. Samtiya M, Aluko RE, Dhewa T. Plant food anti-nutritional factors and their reduction strategies: An overview. *Food Production, Processing and Nutrition.* 2020;2(1). https://doi.org/10.1186/s43014-020-0020-5.

5. Dwyer JT, Wiemer KL, Dary O, et al. Fortification and health: Challenges and opportunities. *Advances in Nutrition.* 2015 Jan 15;6(1):124–31. https://doi.org/10.3945/an.114.007443.

6. Young LM, Pipingas A, White DJ, Gauci S, Scholey A. A systematic review and meta-analysis of B vitamin supplementation on depressive symptoms, anxiety, and stress: Effects on healthy and "at-risk" individuals. *Nutrients.* 2019;11(9):2232. https://doi.org/10.3390/nu11092232.

7. Blasko I, Hinterberger M, Kemmler G, et al. Conversion from mild cognitive impairment to dementia: Influence of folic acid and vitamin B12 use in the VITA cohort. *Journal of Nutrition, Health and Aging.* 2012;16(8):687–94. https://doi.org/10.1007/s12603-012-0051-y; Tangney CC, Aggarwal NT, Li H, et al. Vitamin B12, cognition, and brain MRI measures: A cross-sectional examination. *Neurology.* 2011;77(13):1276–82. https://doi.org/10.1212/WNL.0b013e3182315a33.

8. Mahdavifar B, Hosseinzadeh M, Salehi-Abargouei A, Mirzaei M, Vafa M. Dietary intake of B vitamins and their association with depression, anxiety, and stress symptoms: A cross-sectional, population-based survey. *Journal of Affective Disorders.* 2021;288:92–98. https://doi.org/10.1016/j.jad.2021.03.055.

9. Field DT, Cracknell RO, Eastwood JR, et al. High-dose vitamin B6 supplementation reduces anxiety and strengthens visual surround suppression. *Human Psychopharmacology.* 2022;37(6):e2852. https://doi.org/10.1002/hup.2852.

10. Moore K, Hughes CF, Hoey L, et al. B-vitamins in relation to depression in older adults over 60 years of age: The Trinity Ulster Department of Agriculture (TUDA) Cohort Study. *Journal of the American Medical Directors Association.* 2019;20(5):551–57.e1. https://doi.org/10.1016/j.jamda.2018.11.031.

11. Young LM, Pipingas A, White DJ, Gauci S, Scholey A. A systematic review and meta-analysis of B vitamin supplementation on depressive symptoms, anxiety, and stress: Effects on healthy and "at-risk" individuals. *Nutrients.* 2019;11(9):2232. https://doi.org/10.3390/nu11092232.

12. B Vitamins. The Nutrition Source. Harvard T.H. Chan School of Public Health. Accessed February 16, 2023. https://www.hsph.harvard.edu/nutrition source/vitamins/vitamin-b/.

13. Hemilä H, Chalker E. Vitamin C for preventing and treating the common cold. *Cochrane Database of Systematic Reviews*. 2013;2013(1):CD000980. https://doi.org/10.1002/14651858.CD000980.pub4.

14. Harrison FE, May JM. Vitamin C function in the brain: Vital role of the ascorbate transporter SVCT2. *Free Radical Biology and Medicine*. 2009 Mar 15;46(6):719–30. https://doi.org/10.1016/j.freeradbiomed.2008.12.018.

15. Plevin D, Galletly C. The neuropsychiatric effects of vitamin C deficiency: A systematic review. BMC *Psychiatry*. 2020;20:315. https://doi.org/10.1186 /s12888-020-02730-w.

16. Sim M, Hong S, Jung S, et al. Vitamin C supplementation promotes mental vitality in healthy young adults: Results from a cross-sectional analysis and a randomized, double-blind, placebo-controlled trial. *European Journal of Nutrition*. 2022;61(1):447–59. https://doi.org/10.1007/s00394-021-02656-3.

17. Moritz B, Schmitz AE, Rodrigues ALS, Dafre AL, Cunha MP. The role of vitamin C in stress-related disorders. *Journal of Nutritional Biochemistry*. 2020;85:108459. https://doi.org/10.1016/j.jnutbio.2020.108459.

18. de Oliveira IJ, de Souza VV, Motta V, Da-Silva SL. Effects of oral vitamin C supplementation on anxiety in students: A double-blind, randomized, placebo-controlled trial. *Pakistan Journal of Biological Sciences*. 2015;18(1): 11–18. https://doi.org/10.3923/pjbs.2015.11.18.

19. Vitamin C. The Nutrition Source. Harvard T.H. Chan School of Public Health. Accessed February 16, 2023. https://www.hsph.harvard.edu/nutrition source/vitamin-c/.

20. Ginde AA, Liu MC, Camargo CA Jr. Demographic differences and trends of vitamin D insufficiency in the US population, 1988–2004. *Archives of Internal Medicine*. 2009;169(6):626–32. https://doi.org/10.1001/archinternmed .2008.604.

21. Soni M, Kos K, Lang IA, Jones K, Melzer D, Llewellyn DJ. Vitamin D and cognitive function. *Scandinavian Journal of Clinical and Laboratory Investigation. Supplementum*. 2012;243:79–82. https://doi.org/10.3109/00365513.2012.681969.

22. Anjum I, Jaffery SS, Fayyaz M, Samoo Z, Anjum S. The role of vitamin D in brain health: A mini literature review. *Cureus*. 2018 Jul 10;10(7):e2960. https://doi.org/10.7759/cureus.2960.

23. Cheng YC, Huang YC, Huang WL. The effect of vitamin D supplement on negative emotions: A systematic review and meta-analysis. *Depression and Anxiety*. 2020;37(6):549–64. https://doi.org/10.1002/da.23025.

24. Bičíková M, Dušková M, Vítků J, et al. Vitamin D in anxiety and affective disorders. *Physiological Research.* 2015;64(Suppl 2):S101–S103. https://doi .org/10.33549/physiolres.933082.

25. Zhu C, Zhang Y, Wang T, et al. Vitamin D supplementation improves anxiety but not depression symptoms in patients with vitamin D deficiency. *Brain and Behavior.* 2020;10(11):e01760. https://doi.org/10.1002/brb3.1760.

26. Eid A, Khoja S, AlGhamdi S, et al. Vitamin D supplementation ameliorates severity of generalized anxiety disorder (GAD). *Metabolic Brain Disease.* 2019;34(6):1781–86. https://doi.org/10.1007/s11011-019-00486-1.

27. Armstrong DJ, Meenagh GK, Bickle I, Lee AS, Curran ES, Finch MB. Vitamin D deficiency is associated with anxiety and depression in fibromy-algia. *Clinical Rheumatology.* 2007;26(4):551–54. https://doi.org/10.1007/s10067 -006-0348-5.

28. Norwitz NG, Naidoo U. Nutrition as metabolic treatment for anxiety. *Frontiers in Psychiatry.* 2021;12:598119. https://doi.org/10.3389/fpsyt.2021.598119.

29. La Fata G, Weber P, Mohajeri MH. Effects of vitamin E on cognitive per-formance during ageing and in Alzheimer's disease. *Nutrients.* 2014 Nov 28;6(12):5453–72. https://doi.org/10.3390/nu6125453.

30. Terada Y, Ohashi H, Otani Y, Tokunaga K, Takenaka A. Increased anxiety-like behaviour is an early symptom of vitamin E deficiency that is suppressed by adrenalectomy in rats. *British Journal of Nutrition.* 2021;125(11):1310–19. https://doi.org/10.1017/S0007114520001889.

31. Lee ARYB, Tariq A, Lau G, Tok NWK, Tam WWS, Ho CSH. Vitamin E, alpha-tocopherol, and its effects on depression and anxiety: A systematic review and meta-analysis. *Nutrients.* 2022 Feb 3;14(3):656. https://doi.org /10.3390/nu14030656.

32. Traber MG. Vitamin E inadequacy in humans: Causes and consequences. *Advances in Nutrition.* 2014;5(5):503–14. https://doi.org/10.3945/an.114.006254.

33. Du C, Hsiao PY, Ludy MJ, Tucker RM. Relationships between dairy and calcium intake and mental health measures of higher education students in the United States: Outcomes from moderation analyses. *Nutrients.* 2022 Feb 12;14(4):775. https://doi.org/10.3390/nu14040775.

34. Alkhatatbeh MJ, Khwaileh HN, Abdul-Razzak KK. High prevalence of low dairy calcium intake and association with insomnia, anxiety, depression and musculoskeletal pain in university students from Jordan. *Public Health Nutrition.* 2021;24(7):1778–1786. https://doi.org/10.1017/S1368980020002888.

35. Alkhatatbeh MJ, Abdul-Razzak KK, Khwaileh HN. Poor sleep quality among young adults: The role of anxiety, depression, musculoskeletal pain,

and low dietary calcium intake. *Perspectives in Psychiatric Care.* 2021;57(1): 117–28. https://doi.org/10.1111/ppc.12533.

36. Kim J, Wessling-Resnick M. Iron and mechanisms of emotional behavior. *Journal of Nutritional Biochemistry.* 2014 Nov;25(11):1101–7. https://doi .org/10.1016/j.jnutbio.2014.07.003.

37. Chen MH, Su TP, Chen YS, et al. Association between psychiatric disorders and iron deficiency anemia among children and adolescents: A nationwide population-based study. *BMC Psychiatry.* 2013;13:161. https://doi.org /10.1186/1471-244X-13-161.

38. Shah HE, Bhawnani N, Ethirajulu A, et al. Iron deficiency–induced changes in the hippocampus, corpus striatum, and monoamines levels that lead to anxiety, depression, sleep disorders, and psychotic disorders. *Cureus.* 2021 Sep 20;13(9):e18138. https://doi.org/10.7759/cureus.

39. Kim J, Wessling-Resnick M. Iron and mechanisms of emotional behavior. *Journal of Nutritional Biochemistry.* 2014 Nov;25(11):1101–7. https://doi.org /10.1016/j.jnutbio.2014.07.003.

40. Barbagallo M, Dominguez LJ. Magnesium and type 2 diabetes. *World Journal of Diabetes.* 2015 Aug 25;6(10):1152–57. https://doi.org/10.4239/wjd.v6.i10.1152.

41. Hu L, Bai Y, Hu G, Zhang Y, Han X, Li J. Association of dietary magnesium intake with leukocyte telomere length in United States middle-aged and elderly adults. *Frontiers in Nutrition.* 2022;9:840804. https://doi.org/10.3389 /fnut.2022.840804.

42. Botturi A, Ciappolino V, Delvecchio G, Boscutti A, Viscardi B, Brambilla P. The role and the effect of magnesium in mental disorders: A systematic review. *Nutrients.* 2020 Jun 3;12(6):1661. https://doi.org/10.3390/nu12061661.

43. Jacka FN, Overland S, Stewart R, Tell GS, Bjelland I, Mykletun A. Association between magnesium intake and depression and anxiety in community-dwelling adults: The Hordaland Health Study. *Australian and New Zealand Journal of Psychiatry.* 2009;43(1):45–52. https://doi.org/10.1080 /00048670802534408; Eby GA, Eby KL. Rapid recovery from major depression using magnesium treatment. *Medical Hypotheses.* 2006;67(2):362–70. https://doi.org/10.1016/j.mehy.2006.01.047.

44. Pickering G, Mazur A, Trousselard M, et al. Magnesium status and stress: The vicious circle concept revisited. *Nutrients.* 2020 Nov 28;12(12):3672. https://doi.org/10.3390/nu12123672.

45. Boyle NB, Lawton C, Dye L. The effects of magnesium supplementation on subjective anxiety and stress—a systematic review. *Nutrients.* 2017 Apr 26;9(5):429. https://doi.org/10.3390/nu9050429.

46. Institute of Medicine (US) Standing Committee on the Scientific Evaluation of Dietary Reference Intakes. *Dietary Reference Intakes for Calcium, Phosphorus, Magnesium, Vitamin D, and Fluoride.* Washington, DC: National Academies Press; 1997. Accessed November 20, 2022. http://www.ncbi.nlm .nih.gov/books/NBK109825/.

47. Balachandran RC, Mukhopadhyay S, McBride D, et al. Brain manganese and the balance between essential roles and neurotoxicity. *Journal of Biological Chemistry.* 2020 May 8;295(19):6312–29. https://doi.org/10.1074/jbc .REV119.009453.

48. Takeda A. Manganese action in brain function. *Brain Research. Brain Research Reviews.* 2003;41(1):79–87. https://doi.org/10.1016/s0165-0173(02)00234-5.

49. Ye Q, Kim J. Effect of olfactory manganese exposure on anxiety-related behavior in a mouse model of iron overload hemochromatosis. *Environmental Toxicology and Pharmacology.* 2015 Jul;40(1):333–41. https://doi.org/10 .1016/j.etap.2015.06.016; Bowler RM, Mergler D, Sassine MP, Larribe F, Hudnell K. Neuropsychiatric effects of manganese on mood. *Neurotoxicology.* 1999;20(2–3):367–78.

50. Choi S, Hong DK, Choi BY, Suh SW. Zinc in the brain: Friend or foe? *International Journal of Molecular Sciences.* 2020 Nov 25;21(23):8941. https:// doi.org/10.3390/ijms21238941.

51. Takeda A, Tamano H, Nishio R, Murakami T. Behavioral abnormality induced by enhanced hypothalamo-pituitary-adrenocortical axis activity under dietary zinc deficiency and its usefulness as a model. *International Journal of Molecular Sciences.* 2016 Jul 16;17(7):1149. https://doi.org/10.3390/ijms17071149.

52. Cope EC, Levenson CW. Role of zinc in the development and treatment of mood disorders. *Current Opinion in Clinical Nutrition and Metabolic Care.* 2010;13(6):685–89. https://doi.org/10.1097/MCO.0b013e32833df61a.

53. Russo AJ. Decreased zinc and increased copper in individuals with anxiety. *Nutrition and Metabolic Insights.* 2011;4:1–5. https://doi.org/10.4137/NMI.S6349.

54. Tahmasebi K, Amani R, Nazari Z, Ahmadi K, Moazzen S, Mostafavi SA. Association of mood disorders with serum zinc concentrations in adolescent female students. *Biological Trace Element Research.* 2017;178(2):180–88. https://doi.org/10.1007/s12011-016-0917-7.

55. Anbari-Nogyni Z, Bidaki R, Madadizadeh F, et al. Relationship of zinc status with depression and anxiety among elderly population. *Clinical Nutrition ESPEN.* 2020;37:233–39. https://doi.org/10.1016/j.clnesp.2020.02.008.

56. Li N, Zhao G, Wu W, et al. The efficacy and safety of vitamin C for iron supplementation in adult patients with iron deficiency anemia: A randomized

clinical trial. *JAMA Network Open.* 2020 Nov 2;3(11):e2023644. https://doi .org/10.1001/jamanetworkopen.2020.23644.

57. de Oliveira MR, Silvestrin RB, Mello E, Souza T, Moreira JC. Oxidative stress in the hippocampus, anxiety-like behavior and decreased locomotory and exploratory activity of adult rats: Effects of sub acute vitamin A supplementation at therapeutic doses. *Neurotoxicology.* 2007;28(6):1191–99. https:// doi.org/10.1016/j.neuro.2007.07.008.

58. Gancheva SM, Zhelyazkova-Savova MD. Vitamin K2 improves anxiety and depression but not cognition in rats with metabolic syndrome: A role of blood glucose? *Folia Medica.* 2016;58(4):264–72. https://doi.org/10.1515/folmed -2016-0032.

59. Russo AJ. Decreased zinc and increased copper in individuals with anxiety. *Nutrition and Metabolic Insights.* 2011;4:1–5. https://doi.org/10.4137/NMI .S6349.

60. Portnoy J, Wang J, Wang F, et al. Lower serum selenium concentration associated with anxiety in children. *Journal of Pediatric Nursing.* 2022;63: e121–e126. https://doi.org/10.1016/j.pedn.2021.09.026.

Chapter 9: Bioactives and Herbal Medicine

1. von Känel R, Kasper S, Bondolfi G, et al. Therapeutic effects of Silexan on somatic symptoms and physical health in patients with anxiety disorders: A meta-analysis. *Brain and Behavior.* 2021;11(4):e01997. https://doi.org/10.1002 /brb3.1997.

2. Malcolm BJ, Tallian K. Essential oil of lavender in anxiety disorders: Ready for prime time? *Mental Health Clinician.* 2018 Mar 26;7(4):147–55. https:// doi.org/10.9740/mhc.2017.07.147.

3. Kasper S, Müller WE, Volz HP, Möller HJ, Koch E, Dienel A. Silexan in anxiety disorders: Clinical data and pharmacological background. *World Journal of Biological Psychiatry.* 2018;19(6):412–20. https://www.tandfonline .com/doi/full/10.1080/15622975.2017.1331046.

4. Baldinger P, Höflich AS, Mitterhauser M, et al. Effects of Silexan on the serotonin-1A receptor and microstructure of the human brain: A randomized, placebo-controlled, double-blind, cross-over study with molecular and structural neuroimaging. *International Journal of Neuropsychopharmacology.* 2014;18(4):pyu063. https://doi.org/10.1093/ijnp/pyu063.

5. Panche AN, Diwan AD, Chandra SR. Flavonoids: An overview. *Journal of Nutritional Science.* 2016 Dec 29;5:e47. https://doi.org/10.1017/jns.2016.41. PMID: 28620474; PMCID: PMC5465813.

6. Gomez-Pinilla F, Nguyen TT. Natural mood foods: The actions of polyphenols against psychiatric and cognitive disorders. *Nutritional Neuroscience.* 2012 May;15(3):127–33. https://doi.org/10.1179/1476830511Y.0000000035.

7. Wang X, Yu J, Zhang X. Dietary polyphenols as prospective natural-compound depression treatment from the perspective of intestinal microbiota regulation. *Molecules.* 2022;27(21):7637. https://doi.org/10.3390/molecules27217637.

8. Lin K, Li Y, Toit ED, Wendt L, Sun J. Effects of polyphenol supplementations on improving depression, anxiety, and quality of life in patients with depression. *Frontiers in Psychiatry.* 2021;12:765485. https://doi.org/10.3389/fpsyt.2021.765485.

9. Jia S, Hou Y, Wang D, Zhao X. Flavonoids for depression and anxiety: A systematic review and meta-analysis. *Critical Reviews in Food Science and Nutrition.* Published online April 9, 2022:1–11. https://doi.org/10.1080/10408398.2022.2057914.

10. Ocean N, Howley P, Ensor J. Lettuce be happy: A longitudinal UK study on the relationship between fruit and vegetable consumption and well-being. *Social Science and Medicine.* 2019;222:335–45. https://doi.org/10.1016/j.socscimed.2018.12.017.

11. Subash S, Essa MM, Al-Adawi S, Memon MA, Manivasagam T, Akbar M. Neuroprotective effects of berry fruits on neurodegenerative diseases. *Neural Regeneration Research.* 2014 Aug 15;9(16):1557–66. https://doi.org/10.4103/1673-5374.139483.

12. Porter Y. Antioxidant properties of green broccoli and purple-sprouting broccoli under different cooking conditions. *Bioscience Horizons.* 2012;5(0): hzs004–hzs004. https://doi.org/10.1093/biohorizons/hzs004.

13. Barba FJ, Nikmaram N, Roohinejad S, Khelfa A, Zhu Z, Koubaa M. Bioavailability of glucosinolates and their breakdown products: Impact of processing. *Frontiers in Nutrition.* 2016 Aug 16;3:24. https://doi.org/10.3389/fnut.2016.00024.

14. Manchali S, Chidambara Murthy KN, Patil BS. Crucial facts about health benefits of popular cruciferous vegetables. *Journal of Functional Foods.* 2012;4(1):94–106. https://doi.org/10.1016/j.jff.2011.08.004.

15. Kuran D, Pogorzelska A, Wiktorska K. Breast cancer prevention—is there a future for sulforaphane and its analogs? *Nutrients.* 2020;12(6):1559. https://doi.org/10.3390/nu12061559; Bagheri M, Fazli M, Saeednia S, Gholami Kharanagh M, Ahmadiankia N. Sulforaphane modulates cell migration and expression of β-catenin and epithelial mesenchymal transition markers in breast cancer cells. *Iranian Journal of Public Health.* 2020 Jan;49(1):77–85.

16. Kita M, Uchida S, Yamada K, Ano Y. Anxiolytic effects of theaflavins via dopaminergic activation in the frontal cortex. *Bioscience, Biotechnology, and Biochemistry.* 2019;83(6):1157–62. https://doi.org/10.1080/09168451.2019.1584523.

17. Steptoe A, Gibson EL, Vuononvirta R, et al. The effects of tea on psycho-physiological stress responsivity and post-stress recovery: A randomised double-blind trial. *Psychopharmacology.* 2007;190(1):81–89. https://doi.org/10.1007/s00213-006-0573-2.

18. Yoto A, Fukui N, Kaneda C, et al. Black tea aroma inhibited increase of salivary chromogranin-A after arithmetic tasks. *Journal of Physiological Anthropology.* 2018 Jan 24;37(1):3. https://doi.org/10.1186/s40101-018-0163-0.

19. Dietz C, Dekker M. Effect of green tea phytochemicals on mood and cognition. *Current Pharmaceutical Design.* 2017;23(19):2876–905. https://doi.org/10.2174/1381612823666170105151800.

20. Hidese S, Ogawa S, Ota M, et al. Effects of L-theanine administration on stress-related symptoms and cognitive functions in healthy adults: A randomized controlled trial. *Nutrients.* 2019;11(10):2362. https://doi.org/10.3390/nu11102362.

21. Klevebrant L, Frick A. Effects of caffeine on anxiety and panic attacks in patients with panic disorder: A systematic review and meta-analysis. *General Hospital Psychiatry.* 2022;74:22–31. https://doi.org/10.1016/j.genhosppsych.2021.11.005.

22. Caffeine. The Nutrition Source. Harvard T.H. Chan School of Public Health. https://www.hsph.harvard.edu/nutritionsource/caffeine/.

23. Wu Y, Lu Y, Xie G. Bubble tea consumption and its association with mental health symptoms: An observational cross-sectional study on Chinese young adults. *Journal of Affective Disorders.* 2022;299:620–27. https://doi.org/10.1016/j.jad.2021.12.061.

24. Achour M, Ben Salem I, Ferdousi F, et al. Rosemary tea consumption alters peripheral anxiety and depression biomarkers: A pilot study in limited healthy volunteers. *Journal of the American Nutrition Association.* 2022;41(3):240–49. https://doi.org/10.1080/07315724.2021.1873871.

25. Bazrafshan MR, Jokar M, Shokrpour N, Delam H. The effect of lavender herbal tea on the anxiety and depression of the elderly: A randomized clinical trial. *Complementary Therapies in Medicine.* 2020;50:102393. https://doi.org/10.1016/j.ctim.2020.102393.

26. Mao JJ, Xie SX, Keefe JR, Soeller I, Li QS, Amsterdam JD. Long-term chamomile (*Matricaria chamomilla* L.) treatment for generalized anxiety

disorder: A randomized clinical trial. *Phytomedicine.* 2016;23(14):1735–42. https://doi.org/10.1016/j.phymed.2016.10.012.

27. Piek H, Venter I, Rautenbach F, Marnewick JL. Rooibos herbal tea: An optimal cup and its consumers. *Health SA.* 2019;24:1090. https://doi.org /10.4102/hsag.v24i0.1090.

28. Fusar-Poli L, Gabbiadini A, Ciancio A, Vozza L, Signorelli MS, Aguglia E. The effect of cocoa-rich products on depression, anxiety, and mood: A systematic review and meta-analysis. *Critical Reviews in Food Science and Nutrition.* 2022;62(28):7905–16. https://doi.org/10.1080/10408398.2021.1920570.

29. Martin FP, Rezzi S, Peré-Trepat E, et al. Metabolic effects of dark chocolate consumption on energy, gut microbiota, and stress-related metabolism in free-living subjects. *Journal of Proteome Research.* 2009;8(12):5568–79. https://doi.org/10.1021/pr900607v.

30. Pase MP, Scholey AB, Pipingas A, et al. Cocoa polyphenols enhance positive mood states but not cognitive performance: A randomized, placebo-controlled trial. *Journal of Psychopharmacology.* 2013;27(5):451–58. https:// doi.org/10.1177/0269881112473791.

31. García-Blanco T, Dávalos A, Visioli F. Tea, cocoa, coffee, and affective disorders: Vicious or virtuous cycle? *Journal of Affective Disorders.* 2017;224:61–68. https://doi.org/10.1016/j.jad.2016.11.033.

32. Baum-Baicker C. The psychological benefits of moderate alcohol consumption: A review of the literature. *Drug and Alcohol Dependence.* 1985;15(4):305–22. https://doi.org/10.1016/0376-8716(85)90008-0.

33. Matias JN, Achete G, Campanari GSDS, et al. A systematic review of the antidepressant effects of curcumin: Beyond monoamines theory. *Australian and New Zealand Journal of Psychiatry.* 2021;55(5):451–62. https://doi.org /10.1177/0004867421998795.

34. Esmaily H, Sahebkar A, Iranshahi M, et al. An investigation of the effects of curcumin on anxiety and depression in obese individuals: A randomized controlled trial. *Chinese Journal of Integrative Medicine.* 2015;21(5):332–38. https://doi.org/10.1007/s11655-015-2160-z.

35. Hewlings SJ, Kalman DS. Curcumin: A review of its effects on human health. *Foods.* 2017;6(10):92. https://doi.org/10.3390/foods6100092.

36. Maqbool Z, Arshad MS, Ali A, et al. Potential role of phytochemical extract from saffron in development of functional foods and protection of brain-related disorders. *Oxidative Medicine and Cellular Longevity.* 2022;2022: 6480590. https://doi.org/10.1155/2022/6480590.

37. Marx W, Lane M, Rocks T, et al. Effect of saffron supplementation on symptoms of depression and anxiety: A systematic review and meta-analysis

[published online ahead of print, 2019 May 28]. *Nutrition Reviews.* 2019;nuz023. https://doi.org/10.1093/nutrit/nuz023.

38. Ghasemzadeh Rahbardar M, Hosseinzadeh H. Therapeutic effects of rosemary (*Rosmarinus officinalis* L.) and its active constituents on nervous system disorders. *Iranian Journal of Basic Medical Sciences.* 2020;23(9):1100–1112. https://doi.org/10.22038/ijbms.2020.45269.10541.

39. Jamshidi N, Cohen MM. The clinical efficacy and safety of tulsi in humans: A systematic review of the literature. *Evidence-Based Complementary and Alternative Medicine.* 2017;2017:9217567. https://doi.org/10.1155/2017/9217567.

40. Mechan AO, Fowler A, Seifert N, et al. Monoamine reuptake inhibition and mood-enhancing potential of a specified oregano extract. *British Journal of Nutrition.* 2011;105(8):1150–63. https://doi.org/10.1017/S0007114510004940.

41. Rashrash M, Schommer JC, Brown LM. Prevalence and predictors of herbal medicine use among adults in the United States. *Journal of Patient Experience.* 2017;4(3):108–13. https://doi.org/10.1177/2374373517706612.

42. Bent S. Herbal medicine in the United States: Review of efficacy, safety, and regulation: Grand rounds at University of California, San Francisco Medical Center. *Journal of General Internal Medicine.* 2008 Jun;23(6):854–59. https://doi.org/10.1007/s11606-008-0632-y.

43. Singh N, Bhalla M, de Jager P, Gilca M. An overview on ashwagandha: A Rasayana (rejuvenator) of Ayurveda. *African Journal of Traditional, Complementary, and Alternative Medicines.* 2011;8(5 Suppl):208–13. https://doi.org/10.4314/ajtcam.v8i5S.9.

44. Akhgarjand C, Asoudeh F, Bagheri A, et al. Does ashwagandha supplementation have a beneficial effect on the management of anxiety and stress? A systematic review and meta-analysis of randomized controlled trials. *Phytotherapy Research.* 2022;36(11):4115–24. https://doi.org/10.1002/ptr.7598.

45. Pratte MA, Nanavati KB, Young V, Morley CP. An alternative treatment for anxiety: A systematic review of human trial results reported for the Ayurvedic herb ashwagandha (*Withania somnifera*). *Journal of Alternative and Complementary Medicine.* 2014;20(12):901–8. https://doi.org/10.1089/acm.2014.0177.

46. Lopresti AL, Smith SJ, Malvi H, Kodgule R. An investigation into the stress-relieving and pharmacological actions of an ashwagandha (*Withania somnifera*) extract: A randomized, double-blind, placebo-controlled study. *Medicine.* 2019;98(37):e17186. https://doi.org/10.1097/MD.0000000000017186.

47. Noor-E-Tabassum, Das R, Lami MS, et al. Ginkgo biloba: A treasure of functional phytochemicals with multimedicinal applications. *Evidence-Based Complementary and Alternative Medicine.* 2022;2022:8288818. https://doi.org/10.1155/2022/8288818.

48. Woelk H, Arnoldt KH, Kieser M, Hoerr R. Ginkgo biloba special extract EGb 761 in generalized anxiety disorder and adjustment disorder with anxious mood: A randomized, double-blind, placebo-controlled trial. *Journal of Psychiatric Research.* 2007;41(6):472–80. https://doi.org/10.1016/j.jpsychires.2006.05.004.

49. Lee S, Rhee DK. Effects of ginseng on stress-related depression, anxiety, and the hypothalamic-pituitary-adrenal axis. *Journal of Ginseng Research.* 2017 Oct;41(4):589–94. https://doi.org/10.1016/j.jgr.2017.01.010.

50. Sarris J, Byrne GJ, Bousman CA, et al. Kava for generalised anxiety disorder: A 16-week double-blind, randomised, placebo-controlled study. *Australian and New Zealand Journal of Psychiatry.* 2020;54(3):288–97. https://doi.org/10.1177/0004867419891246; Sarris J, Stough C, Bousman CA, et al. Kava in the treatment of generalized anxiety disorder: A double-blind, randomized, placebo-controlled study. *Journal of Clinical Psychopharmacology.* 2013;33(5):643–48. https://doi.org/10.1097/JCP.0b013e318291be67.

51. Ooi SL, Henderson P, Pak SC. Kava for generalized anxiety disorder: A review of current evidence. *Journal of Alternative and Complementary Medicine.* 2018;24(8):770–80. https://doi.org/10.1089/acm.2018.0001.

52. Janda K, Wojtkowska K, Jakubczyk K, Antoniewicz J, Skonieczna-Żydecka K. *Passiflora incarnata* in neuropsychiatric disorders — a systematic review. *Nutrients.* 2020 Dec 19;12(12):3894. https://doi.org/10.3390/nu12123894.

53. Panossian A, Wikman G. Effects of adaptogens on the central nervous system and the molecular mechanisms associated with their stress-protective activity. *Pharmaceuticals.* 2010 Jan 19;3(1):188–224. https://doi.org/10.3390/ph3010188.

54. Bystritsky A, Kerwin L, Feusner JD. A pilot study of *Rhodiola rosea* (Rhodax) for generalized anxiety disorder (GAD). *Journal of Alternative and Complementary Medicine.* 2008;14(2):175–80. https://doi.org/10.1089/acm.2007.7117.

55. Cropley M, Banks AP, Boyle J. The effects of *Rhodiola rosea* L. extract on anxiety, stress, cognition and other mood symptoms. *Phytotherapy Research.* 2015;29(12):1934–39. https://doi.org/10.1002/ptr.5486.

56. Sharpe L, Sinclair J, Kramer A, de Manincor M, Sarris J. Cannabis, a cause for anxiety? A critical appraisal of the anxiogenic and anxiolytic properties. *Journal of Translational Medicine.* 2020;18(1):374. https://doi.org/10.1186/s12967-020-02518-2.

Chapter 10: An Antianxiety Shopping Trip

1. Jin H, Lu Y. Evaluating consumer nutrition environment in food deserts and food swamps. *International Journal of Environmental Research and Public Health.* 2021 Mar 7;18(5):2675. https://doi.org/10.3390/ijerph18052675.

2. Bergmans RS, Sadler RC, Wolfson JA, Jones AD, Kruger D. Moderation of the association between individual food security and poor mental health by the local food environment among adult residents of Flint, Michigan. *Health Equity.* 2019 Jun 14;3(1):264–74. https://doi.org/10.1089/heq.2018.0103.

3. Vigar V, Myers S, Oliver C, Arellano J, Robinson S, Leifert C. A systematic review of organic versus conventional food consumption: Is there a measurable benefit on human health? *Nutrients.* 2019 Dec 18;12(1):7. https://doi.org/10.3390/nu12010007.

4. Glibowski P. Organic food and health. *Roczniki Państwowego Zakładu Higieny.* 2020;71(2):131–36. https://doi.org/10.32394/rpzh.2020.0110.

5. Zeni ALB, Camargo A, Dalmagro AP. Lutein prevents corticosterone-induced depressive-like behavior in mice with the involvement of antioxidant and neuroprotective activities. *Pharmacology, Biochemistry, and Behavior.* 2019;179:63–72. https://doi.org/10.1016/j.pbb.2019.02.004.

6. Sedlak TW, Nucifora LG, Koga M, et al. Sulforaphane augments glutathione and influences brain metabolites in human subjects: A clinical pilot study. *Molecular Neuropsychiatry.* 2018;3(4):214–22. https://doi.org/10.1159/000487639.

7. Cheng L, Pan GF, Sun XB, Huang YX, Peng YS, Zhou LY. Evaluation of anxiolytic-like effect of aqueous extract of asparagus stem in mice. *Evidence-Based Complementary and Alternative Medicine.* 2013;2013:587260. https://doi.org/10.1155/2013/587260.

8. Bhaswant M, Shanmugam DK, Miyazawa T, Abe C, Miyazawa T. Microgreens—a comprehensive review of bioactive molecules and health benefits. *Molecules.* 2023;28(2):867. https://doi.org/10.3390/molecules28020867.

9. Deepika, Maurya PK. Health benefits of quercetin in age-related diseases. *Molecules.* 2022;27(8):2498. https://doi.org/10.3390/molecules27082498.

10. Wang L, Tao L, Hao L, et al. A moderate-fat diet with one avocado per day increases plasma antioxidants and decreases the oxidation of small, dense LDL in adults with overweight and obesity: A randomized controlled trial. *Journal of Nutrition.* 2020;150(2):276–84. https://doi.org/10.1093/jn/nxz231.

11. Bouzari A, Holstege D, Barrett DM. Vitamin retention in eight fruits and vegetables: A comparison of refrigerated and frozen storage. *Journal of Agricultural and Food Chemistry.* 2015;63(3):957–62. https://doi.org/10.1021/jf5058793.

12. Jensen IJ, Eilertsen KE, Otnæs CHA, Mæhre HK, Elvevoll EO. An update on the content of fatty acids, dioxins, PCBs and heavy metals in farmed, escaped and wild Atlantic salmon (*Salmo salar* L.) in Norway. *Foods.* 2020;9(12):1901. https://doi.org/10.3390/foods9121901.

13. Dawson P, Al-Jeddawi W, Remington N. Effect of freezing on the shelf life of salmon. *International Journal of Food Science*. 2018 Aug 12;2018:1686121. https://doi.org/10.1155/2018/1686121.

14. Norberg J, Blenckner T, Cornell SE, Petchey OL, Hillebrand H. Failures to disagree are essential for environmental science to effectively influence policy development. *Ecology Letters*. 2022 May;25(5):1075–93. https://doi.org /10.1111/ele.13984.

15. Jarmul S, Dangour AD, Green R, Liew Z, Haines A, Scheelbeek PF. Climate change mitigation through dietary change: A systematic review of empirical and modelling studies on the environmental footprints and health effects of "sustainable diets." *Environmental Research Letters*. 2020 Dec 22;15:123014. https://doi.org/10.1088/1748-9326/abc2f7.

16. Provenza FD, Kronberg SL, Gregorini P. Is grassfed meat and dairy better for human and environmental health? *Frontiers in Nutrition*. 2019;6:26. https://doi.org/10.3389/fnut.2019.00026.

17. Chazelas E, Pierre F, Druesne-Pecollo N, et al. Nitrites and nitrates from food additives and natural sources and cancer risk: Results from the NutriNet-Santé cohort. *International Journal of Epidemiology*. 2022;51(4):1106–19. https://doi.org/10.1093/ije/dyac046.

18. Messina M, Duncan A, Messina V, Lynch H, Kiel J, Erdman JW Jr. The health effects of soy: A reference guide for health professionals. *Frontiers in Nutrition*. 2022;9:970364. https://doi.org/10.3389/fnut.2022.970364.

19. Boutas I, Kontogeorgi A, Dimitrakakis C, Kalantaridou SN. Soy isoflavones and breast cancer risk: A meta-analysis. *In Vivo*. 2022 Mar–Apr;36(2):556–62. https://doi.org/10.21873/invivo.12737.

20. Ota A, Yamamoto A, Kimura S, et al. Rational identification of a novel soy-derived anxiolytic-like undecapeptide acting via gut-brain axis after oral administration. *Neurochemistry International*. 2017;105:51–57. https://doi.org/10.1016/j.neuint.2016.12.020.

21. Fernandez ML, Murillo AG. Is there a correlation between dietary and blood cholesterol? Evidence from epidemiological data and clinical interventions. *Nutrients*. 2022 May 23;14(10):2168. https://doi.org/10.3390/nu14102168.

22. Drouin-Chartier JP, Chen S, Li Y, et al. Egg consumption and risk of cardiovascular disease: Three large prospective US cohort studies, systematic review, and updated meta-analysis. *BMJ*. 2020;368:m513. https://doi.org /10.1136/bmj.m513.

23. Alothman M, Hogan SA, Hennessy D, et al. The "grass-fed" milk story: Understanding the impact of pasture feeding on the composition and quality of bovine milk. *Foods*. 2019 Aug 17;8(8):350. https://doi.org/10.3390/foods8080350.

24. Jaatinen N, Korpela R, Poussa T, et al. Effects of daily intake of yoghurt enriched with bioactive components on chronic stress responses: A double-blinded randomized controlled trial. *International Journal of Food Sciences and Nutrition.* 2014;65(4):507–14. https://doi.org/10.3109/09637486.2014.880669; Sousa RJM, Baptista JAB, Silva CCG. Consumption of fermented dairy products is associated with lower anxiety levels in Azorean University students. *Frontiers in Nutrition.* 2022;9:930949. https://doi.org/10.3389/fnut.2022.930949.

25. Hodges C, Archer F, Chowdhury M, et al. Method of food preparation influences blood glucose response to a high-carbohydrate meal: A randomised cross-over trial. *Foods.* 2019 Dec 25;9(1):23. https://doi.org/10.3390/foods9010023.

26. Devaraj RD, Reddy CK, Xu B. Health-promoting effects of konjac glucomannan and its practical applications: A critical review. *International Journal of Biological Macromolecules.* 2019;126:273–81. https://doi.org/10.1016/j.ijbiomac.2018.12.203.

27. Sugiyama M, Tang AC, Wakaki Y, Koyama W. Glycemic index of single and mixed meal foods among common Japanese foods with white rice as a reference food. *European Journal of Clinical Nutrition.* 2003;57(6):743–52. https://doi.org/10.1038/sj.ejcn.1601606.

28. 10 of the Worst Foods for Blood Sugar—According to CGM Data. Levels Health. June 18, 2022. Updated November 2, 2022. Accessed February 22, 2023. https://www.levelshealth.com/blog/10-of-the-worst-foods-for-blood-sugar-according-to-cgm-data.

29. Flores M, Saravia C, Vergara CE, Avila F, Valdés H, Ortiz-Viedma J. Avocado oil: Characteristics, properties, and applications. *Molecules.* 2019 Jun 10;24(11):2172. https://doi.org/10.3390/molecules24112172.

30. Leeuwendaal NK, Stanton C, O'Toole PW, Beresford TP. Fermented foods, health and the gut microbiome. *Nutrients.* 2022;14(7):1527. https://doi.org/10.3390/nu14071527.

31. Haghighatdoost F, Feizi A, Esmaillzadeh A, et al. Drinking plain water is associated with decreased risk of depression and anxiety in adults: Results from a large cross-sectional study. *World Journal of Psychiatry.* 2018;8(3):88–96. https://doi.org/10.5498/wjp.v8.i3.88.

32. Kaur S, Christian H, Cooper MN, Francis J, Allen K, Trapp G. Consumption of energy drinks is associated with depression, anxiety, and stress in young adult males: Evidence from a longitudinal cohort study. *Depression and Anxiety.* 2020;37(11):1089–98. https://doi.org/10.1002/da.23090.

33. Klevebrant L, Frick A. Effects of caffeine on anxiety and panic attacks in patients with panic disorder: A systematic review and meta-analysis. *General*

Hospital Psychiatry. 2022;74:22–31. https://doi.org/10.1016/j.genhosppsych
.2021.11.005.

34. Torvik FA, Rosenström TH, Gustavson K, et al. Explaining the association
    between anxiety disorders and alcohol use disorder: A twin study. *Depression and Anxiety.* 2019;36(6):522–32. https://doi.org/10.1002/da.22886.

35. Schleider JL, Ye F, Wang F, Hipwell AE, Chung T, Sartor C. Longitudinal
    reciprocal associations between anxiety, depression, and alcohol use in
    adolescent girls. *Alcoholism, Clinical and Experimental Research.* 2019;43(1):
    98–107. https://doi.org/10.1111/acer.13913.

36. Gibson-Smith D, Bot M, Brouwer IA, Visser M, Giltay EJ, Penninx BWJH.
    Association of food groups with depression and anxiety disorders. *European
    Journal of Nutrition.* 2020;59(2):767–78. https://doi.org/10.1007/s00394-019
    -01943-4.

37. Johnston M, McBride M, Dahiya D, Owusu-Apenten R, Nigam PS. Antibacterial activity of manuka honey and its components: An overview.
    AIMS Microbiology. 2018;4(4):655–64. https://doi.org/10.3934/microbiol
    .2018.4.655.

38. Callahan A. Do I need to avoid dark chocolate now? *New York Times.*
    February 9, 2023. Accessed February 23, 2023. https://www.nytimes.com
    /2023/02/09/well/eat/dark-chocolate-metal-lead.html.

Chapter 11: The Six Pillars to Calm Your Mind

1. Buettner D, Skemp S. Blue Zones: Lessons from the world's longest lived.
   American Journal of Lifestyle Medicine. 2016 Jul 7;10(5):318–21. https://doi
   .org/10.1177/1559827616637066.

2. Marston HR, Niles-Yokum K, Silva PA. A commentary on Blue Zones®: A
   critical review of age-friendly environments in the 21st century and beyond.
   International Journal of Environmental Research and Public Health. 2021 Jan
   19;18(2):837. https://doi.org/10.3390/ijerph18020837.

3. Heath C, Lopez NV, Seeton V, Sutliffe JT. Blue Zones–based worksite
   nutrition intervention: Positive impact on employee wellbeing. *Frontiers in
   Nutrition.* 2022 Feb 11;9:795387. https://doi.org/10.3389/fnut.2022.795387.

4. Buettner D, Skemp S. Blue Zones: Lessons from the world's longest lived.
   American Journal of Lifestyle Medicine. 2016 Jul 7;10(5):318–21. https://doi
   .org/10.1177/1559827616637066.

Chapter 12: Building Your Antianxiety Eating Plan

1. Altomare R, Cacciabaudo F, Damiano G, et al. The Mediterranean diet: A
   history of health. *Iranian Journal of Public Health.* 2013 May 1;42(5):449–57.

2. Ventriglio A, Sancassiani F, Contu MP, et al. Mediterranean diet and its benefits on health and mental health: A literature review. *Clinical Practice and Epidemiology in Mental Health*. 2020 Jul 30;16(Suppl 1):156–64. https://doi.org/10.2174/1745017902016010156.

3. Merra G, Noce A, Marrone G, et al. Influence of Mediterranean diet on human gut microbiota. *Nutrients*. 2020;13(1):7. https://doi.org/10.3390/nu13010007.

4. Merra G, Noce A, Marrone G, et al. Influence of Mediterranean diet on human gut microbiota. *Nutrients*. 2020;13(1):7. https://doi.org/10.3390/nu13010007.

5. Yin W, Löf M, Chen R, Hultman CM, Fang F, Sandin S. Mediterranean diet and depression: A population-based cohort study. *International Journal of Behavioral Nutrition and Physical Activity*. 2021;18(1):153. https://doi.org/10.1186/s12966-021-01227-3.

6. Pallauf K, Giller K, Huebbe P, Rimbach G. Nutrition and healthy ageing: Calorie restriction or polyphenol-rich "MediterrAsian" diet? *Oxidative Medicine and Cellular Longevity*. 2013;2013:707421. https://doi.org/10.1155/2013/707421.

7. Włodarczyk A, Cubała WJ, Wielewicka A. Ketogenic diet: A dietary modification as an anxiolytic approach? *Nutrients*. 2020 Dec 14;12(12):3822. https://doi.org/10.3390/nu12123822. PMID: 33327540; PMCID: PMC7765029.

8. Sullivan PG, Rippy NA, Dorenbos K, Concepcion RC, Agarwal AK, Rho JM. The ketogenic diet increases mitochondrial uncoupling protein levels and activity. *Annals of Neurology*. 2004;55(4):576–80. https://doi.org/10.1002/ana.20062.

9. Tillery EE, Ellis KD, Threatt TB, Reyes HA, Plummer CS, Barney LR. The use of the ketogenic diet in the treatment of psychiatric disorders. *Mental Health Clinician*. 2021;11(3):211–19. https://doi.org/10.9740/mhc.2021.05.211.

10. Tidman M. Effects of a ketogenic diet on symptoms, biomarkers, depression, and anxiety in Parkinson's disease: A case study. *Cureus*. 2022 Mar 31;14(3):e23684. https://doi.org/10.7759/cureus.23684.

11. Paoli A, Mancin L, Bianco A, Thomas E, Mota JF, Piccini F. Ketogenic diet and microbiota: Friends or enemies? *Genes*. 2019;10(7):534. https://doi.org/10.3390/genes10070534.

12. Masood W, Annamaraju P, Uppaluri KR. Ketogenic Diet. StatPearls. June 11, 2022. https://www.ncbi.nlm.nih.gov/books/NBK499830/.

13. Schutz Y, Montani J, Dulloo AG. Low-carbohydrate ketogenic diets in body weight control: A recurrent plaguing issue of fad diets? *Obesity Reviews*. 2021;22(S2). https://doi.org/10.1111/obr.13195.

14. Vasim I, Majeed CN, DeBoer MD. Intermittent fasting and metabolic health. *Nutrients*. 2022 Jan 31;14(3):631. https://doi.org/10.3390/nu14030631. PMID: 35276989; PMCID: PMC8839325.

15. Berthelot E, Etchecopar-Etchart D, Thellier D, Lancon C, Boyer L, Fond G. Fasting interventions for stress, anxiety and depressive symptoms: A systematic review and meta-analysis. *Nutrients.* 2021 Nov 5;13(11):3947. https://doi.org/10.3390/nu13113947.

16. Gudden J, Arias Vasquez A, Bloemendaal M. The effects of intermittent fasting on brain and cognitive function. *Nutrients.* 2021 Sep 10;13(9):3166. https://doi.org/10.3390/nu13093166.

17. Bjornsson AS, Didie ER, Phillips KA. Body dysmorphic disorder. *Dialogues in Clinical Neuroscience.* 2010;12(2):221–32. https://doi.org/10.31887 /DCNS.2010.12.2/abjornsson.

18. Scarff JR. Orthorexia nervosa: An obsession with healthy eating. *Federal Practitioner.* 2017 Jun;34(6):36–39. PMID: 30766283; PMCID: PMC6370446.

19. Smith AR, Zuromski KL, Dodd DR. Eating disorders and suicidality: What we know, what we don't know, and suggestions for future research. *Current Opinion in Psychology.* 2018;22:63–67. https://doi.org/10.1016/j.copsyc.2017 .08.023.

20. Yılmaz MN, Dundar C. The relationship between orthorexia nervosa, anxiety, and self-esteem: A cross-sectional study in Turkish faculty members. *BMC Psychology.* 2022;10(1):82. https://doi.org/10.1186/s40359-022-00796-7.

21. Lee SD, Kellow NJ, Choi TST, Huggins CE. Assessment of dietary acculturation in East Asian populations: A scoping review. *Advances in Nutrition.* 2020;12(3):865–86. https://doi.org/10.1093/advances/nmaa127.

22. Neumark-Sztainer D, Wall M, Guo J, Story M, Haines J, Eisenberg M. Obesity, disordered eating, and eating disorders in a longitudinal study of adolescents: How do dieters fare 5 years later? *Journal of the American Dietetic Association.* 2006;106(4):559–68. https://doi.org/10.1016/j.jada.2006.01.003.

23. Stice E, Burger K, Yokum S. Caloric deprivation increases responsivity of attention and reward brain regions to intake, anticipated intake, and images of palatable foods. *Neuroimage.* 2013;67:322–30. https://doi.org/10 .1016/j.neuroimage.2012.11.028.

24. Hussenoeder FS, Conrad I, Engel C, et al. Analyzing the link between anxiety and eating behavior as a potential pathway to eating-related health outcomes. *Scientific Reports.* 2021;11:14717. https://doi.org/10.1038/s41598 -021-94279-1; Lloyd EC, Haase AM, Verplanken B. Anxiety and the development and maintenance of anorexia nervosa: Protocol for a systematic review. *Systematic Reviews.* 2018;7:14. https://doi.org/10.1186/s13643-018-0685-x.

25. Mestre ZL, Melhorn SJ, Askren MK, et al. Effects of anxiety on caloric intake and satiety-related brain activation in women and men. *Psychosomatic Medicine.* 2016;78(4):454–64. https://doi.org/10.1097/PSY.0000000000000299.

Index

Index

About the Author

Uma Naidoo, MD, is a board-certified psychiatrist (Harvard Medical School), professional chef (Cambridge School of Culinary Arts), and nutrition specialist (Cornell University). She is currently the director of Nutritional and Lifestyle Psychiatry at Massachusetts General Hospital, where she consults on nutritional interventions for the psychiatrically and medically ill; is director of Nutritional Psychiatry at the Massachusetts General Hospital Academy; and has a private practice in Newton, Massachusetts. She also teaches at the Cambridge School of Culinary Arts. Dr. Naidoo speaks frequently at conferences at Harvard, for Goop audiences, at the New York City Jewish Community Center, and at Ivy Boston. She blogs for *Harvard Health* and *Psychology Today* and has just completed a unique video cooking series for the Massachusetts General Hospital Academy that teaches nutritional psychiatry using culinary techniques in the kitchen. She has been asked by the American Psychiatric Association to author the first text in the area of nutritional psychiatry. Baking is one of her true passions, in addition to savory cooking.